KU-649-231

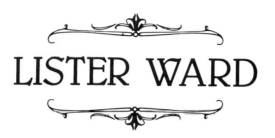

LISTER WARD

Martin Goldman

(Deceased: Formerly of BBC Radio Scotland, Edinburgh)

Adam Hilger
Bristol and Boston

© Mrs Frances Goldman 1987

All rights reserved. No part of this publication may be reproduced, stored in a retrieval system or transmitted in any form or by any means, electronic, mechanical, photocopying, recording or otherwise, without the prior permission of the publisher.

British Library Cataloguing in Publication Data

Lister Ward
  1. Royal Infirmary of Edinburgh——History
  2. Tuberculosis——Hospitals and
     sanatoriums——Scotland——Edinburgh
  (Lothian)   3. Tuberculosis——Personal
  narratives
  I. Goldman, Martin
  362.1'96995'00922   RC309.5.G7

  ISBN 0-85274-562-1

Consultant Editor: **Professor A J Meadows**,
University of Leicester

Published under the Adam Hilger imprint by
IOP Publishing Ltd
Techno House, Redcliffe Way, Bristol BS1 6NX, England
PO Box 230, Accord, MA 02018, USA

Typeset by BC Typesetting, Bristol BS15 6PJ

Printed in Great Britain by J W Arrowsmith Ltd, Bristol

LISTER WARD

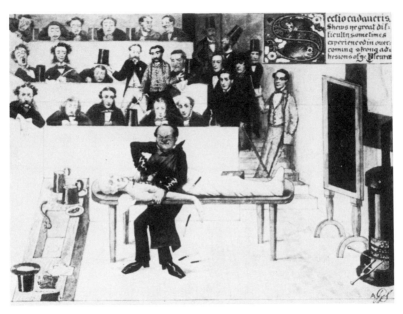

The popular image of a surgical operation from pre-anaesthetic days. (Courtesy of Professor Sir Alastair Currie, University of Edinburgh Medical School)

IN MEMORIAM

CONTENTS

PREFACE

This book is about what it was like to be a patient in a Victorian hospital, the Edinburgh Royal Infirmary, at the time when Joseph Lister was pioneering the use of antiseptics.

Much has already been written about this period, but most first-hand accounts have come from doctors who had been Lister's students and were written in the twentieth century through a mellow haze of hero worship. One such book is *Lister as I Knew Him* by John Rudd Leeson which, while neither more nor less hagiographical than the other accounts, is perhaps a little more lively. Extracts from it are used here to amplify, but more interestingly to contrast with, two mostly unpublished accounts of everyday hospital life of this period from the wrong side of the blanket – from patients who were on the receiving end of antiseptic surgery. The two patients, William Ernest Henley and Margaret Catherine Sarah Mathewson, were both operated on by Lister for tuberculosis.

William Henley was an intimate friend of Robert Louis Stevenson and later became the editor of *The National Observer*, perhaps the most influential literary magazine of the period. While in hospital he wrote a sequence of poems and also a series of far less formal letters to a friend in London. Margaret Mathewson achieved no renown in the literary world. But in hospital she wrote letters to her family with a truly Victorian prolificacy, and then wrote a quite remarkable *Sketch* – a reconstructed journal of her eight-month stay – when she returned home.

The two individual stories reflect the universal experience of countless Victorian patients. This would often begin with a long and uncomfortable journey to the hospital, where the first major hurdle had to be surmounted: admission was at the discretion of the Professor of Surgery. If admitted, but not requiring urgent treatment, the patient would next be lectured on for the benefit of medical students. The operation followed, but even if it were successful, and even if the patient recovered from the chloroform, there came next the terrible risk of post-operative infection. If this too were overcome, there was then a period of enforced idleness and convalescence which, for tuberculosis patients, could last for months.

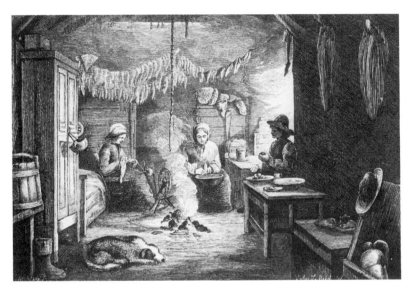

The interior of a Shetland cottage. The illustration comes from a book published in 1869 and the text reads: '. . . a fair sample of the Shetland cottage and contains most of the articles of furniture peculiar to the country – the tall wooden press, long resting-chair or sofa, box-beds, anker-kettle, *daffach*, arm chairs and spinning wheels. The fire is in the middle of the floor and rows of piltocks, and *hoes* or dog-fish, are hung across the roof to obtain the benefit of the "reek".' (National Library of Scotland)

The main body of the text follows this sequence of events in chronological order. Even though Henley and Mathewson were not in hospital at the same time and never met each other, their

x

accounts are so vivid, so gripping and dovetail together so well
that they have simply been put together with a minimum of
explanatory text to build a mosaic of their experience in a
Victorian hospital.

INTRODUCTION

William Henley's and Margaret Mathewson's accounts of hospital life derive a significance beyond their individual testaments of hope and survival from the period in which they took place: for at that time the Edinburgh Royal Infirmary was witnessing the birth of modern medicine. Until Lister and antiseptic surgery, a hospital had been a place to go to be killed rather than cured, as John Rudd Leeson wrote:

> I remember a sturdy young countryman coming as an out-patient and blushingly telling the assistant surgeon that he was about to be married, and that his sweetheart had alluded to the fact that his nose was too much to one side, could it not be straightened? He had heard of the wonderful things that were done in London hospitals! He was admitted, the septum was straightened, and in five days he was lying upon the post-mortem table, dead of acute sepsis![1]

In hospitals lurked the various bacteria that made surgical wounds turn septic and caused diseases such as septicaemia or pyaemia (serious forms of blood poisoning), erysipelas (inflammation of the skin) and gangrene. These diseases were so prevalent in hospitals that they were collectively known as 'hospitalism'.

The situation was no better in Edinburgh, then one of the leading medical centres in the world. The Royal Infirmary there had been founded in 1729, both as a charitable act to provide hospital care for the needy sick (the wealthy were then and for many years afterwards treated in their own homes) and as a resource for clinical teaching. Three years earlier, in 1726,

1

Edinburgh's Town Council had decided to set up a medical faculty in the University. This was partly a financial move to stop Scottish students studying abroad (particularly at Leyden in Holland) and taking their money *out* of the country, and to attract foreign students and their money *in*.

With the close connections between the two institutions, the practice of clinical teaching developed. This meant using real patients to exemplify diseases, and teaching students diagnosis in real situations rather than through textbooks, which was what happened elsewhere. The professors were paid rather small salaries, but every student who attended a course of lectures had to pay his teacher a class fee. Some say that this inducement to lecture well played a large part in Edinburgh's success, for under a formidable series of teachers, and by a liberal admission policy and its relative cheapness, Edinburgh became the foremost medical centre in the English-speaking world in the eighteenth century, attracting many students from America, England and Ireland.

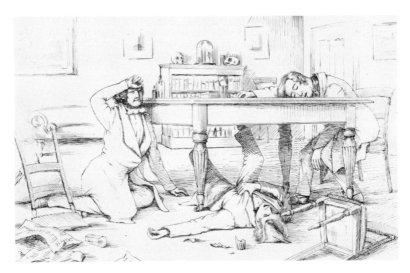

Sir James Young Simpson, Dr Thomas Keith and Dr James Matthews Duncan experiencing the effects of chloroform on 4 November 1857. (Wellcome Institute Library, London)

2

The nineteenth century saw an expansion in university medical education in England (largely staffed by Edinburgh graduates) and a decline in Edinburgh's absolute medical monopoly. None the less, Edinburgh still contributed many charismatic figures to medical history. One of these was Sir James Young Simpson, Professor of Midwifery and a man of great ability and far-ranging interests not only in the whole of medicine but also in history and archaeology.

Simpson was responsible for the introduction of chloroform as an anaesthetic. Ether had been the first anaesthetic tried, successfully, in America in October 1846. It took two months before Britain heard of this remarkable discovery, and ether was promptly given a public trial by Robert Liston (another Edinburgh man) at University College, London. Lister, as a young medical student, was in the audience to hear Liston's comment: 'This Yankee dodge, gentlemen, beats mesmerism hollow.'

Simpson soon tried ether as a means of reducing pain in childbirth. Although it worked well, he began a search for other, possibly better, agents and became involved with a group of friends in inhaling all manner of volatile liquids to see what happened. These 'proto-glue-sniffers' got the occasional 'high', seriously damaged their health and discovered chloroform. In a letter, Simpson describes how he was quite carried away by the great moment:

> On the first occasion on which I detected the anaesthetic effects of chloroform, the scene was an odd one. I had had the chloroform beside me for several days, but it seemed so unlikely a liquid to produce results of any kind, that it was laid aside, and on searching for another object among some loose paper, after coming home very late one night, my hand chanced to fall upon it, and I poured some of the fluid into tumblers before my assistants, Dr Keith and Dr Duncan, and myself. Before sitting down to supper, we all inhaled the fluid, and were all 'under the mahogany' in a trice, to my wife's consternation and alarm.[2]

Even after the acceptance of chloroform, the dedicated

3

researchers resolutely continued sniffing:

> Among other experiments, Dr Simpson had got an
> effervescing drink prepared with chloric ether in aerated
> water. At a dinner party this was brought forward and
> tried, pronounced to be very pleasant, but rather heady.
> The butler took the remains of this new beverage down-
> stairs and gave it to the cook, saying it was champagne.
> Shortly after drinking it, she fell on the floor insensible.
> The butler rushed into the dining-room, saying 'For God's
> sake, sir, come down; I've pushioned [poisoned] the cook.'
> Dr S with some others ran down-stairs, and found their
> patient lying on the floor, snoring heavily. The butler
> explained that he had given her a glass of 'the new
> champagne chlory'. As there was no danger, the incident
> created a hearty laugh.[3]

The use of anaesthetics in surgery meant that the patient
stayed still for the duration of the operation. Thus, more
delicate surgery could be performed. Previously, the writhings
of the patient and the postoperative shock that extreme pain
caused had placed a premium on a surgeon's speed. It was, in
fact, Robert Liston who was generally regarded as one of the
fastest in the business. He could amputate a leg, including
sawing through the thigh bone, in 29 seconds. He once,
reputedly, amputated a leg, took off two of his assistant's fingers
and cut off the tail of an on-looker's frock coat, all in the same
operation! A surgeon required a good eye, steely fingers and an
obliviousness to the suffering of others. There did not seem to be
any requirements on intelligence. Traditionally, surgery had
been a fairly low-grade occupation; surgeons had been allied
with barbers as a guild.

Anaesthetics ended that chapter of surgical history, for the
surgeon could now be a careful, methodical operator. Actually,
it threw into sharp relief the very primitive state of medicine at
the time. There had been great advances in anatomy, in the
understanding of the way the various parts of the body articulated, but no corresponding advances in understanding how to
cure those parts when they went wrong. There was vaccination
for smallpox, quinine for malaria and that was about it. (And

that was where it remained, despite medical bombast, frock coats and stiff collars until sulpha drugs in the 1930s!) The only hope was for a surgeon to cut a diseased organ out. Previously, surgeons had been limited to superficial operations that were quick. Now they could probe deeper, but this invariably left larger surgical wounds and therefore a more propitious site for infection to flourish. Whenever they tried anything more ambitious, the operational wounds became septic and the patient died. Nothing was understood of the nature of infection, and without any theoretical structure to guide their minds it was exceedingly difficult for doctors to develop a coherent, scientific approach to the problem of curing disease.

The first breakthrough was made by James Young Simpson who took a revolutionary, objective, *statistical* look at disease. His work here was far more profound and significant than his discovery of chloroform. As an obstetrician, his first interest was in the incidence of puerperal fever. This is now understood to be an infection caused by bacteria invading the body through the damaged womb of a woman after childbirth. Then, it was a mysterious disease, the incidence of which varied from place to place but in some hospitals it killed more than one mother in ten. He found that it was generally far safer to have a baby at home than in a hospital.

Simpson then applied his methods to surgical operations and earned the undying hatred of the surgical fraternity. He realized that there were similarities between puerperal fever and the disease that so frequently followed surgery. He therefore applied his statistical techniques to amputations. Surgeons were rather complacent about amputations, being quick, peripheral operations which they understood, and yet the death rate after amputation was horrendous. It varied from hospital to hospital and from year to year, but it was uniformly high: in Edinburgh and Glasgow it stood at around 40 per cent. As late as 1874, John Eric Erichsen, Professor of Surgery at University College, London, who had taught Lister but never accepted the revolution that his star pupil initiated, could write: 'a mortality of from 24 to 26 per cent may be considered very satisfactory.' In the army the mortality was from 70 to 90 per cent.[4]

When Simpson analysed the amputation data, he obtained the same result as he had done for puerperal fever, namely that hospitals killed patients, which led him to coin the name 'hospitalism' for post-surgical septic disease. He found that of 2,089 patients having amputations performed in hospital, 855 (approximately 41 per cent) died; of 2,098 patients having amputations performed *outside* hospital, 226 (11 per cent) died. Simpson wrote: 'A man laid on the operating table in one of our surgical hospitals is exposed to more chances of death than was the English Soldier on the field of Waterloo.'[5] Simpson's results made many hospital administrators think about 'disinfecting' their persistently infected wards, though only in Lincoln, it would appear, did the Governors carry the analysis through to the logical conclusion that Simpson saw as the only ultimately satisfactory solution.

> Once a hospital has become incurably pyaemia-stricken, it is as impossible to disinfect it by any known hygenic means, as it would to disinfect an old cheese of the maggots which have been generated in it. There is in these extreme cases, only one remedy left, that remedy which the Governors and Staff of the Lincoln Country Hospital have so generously, so disinterestly, so nobly resolved on – the demolition of the infected fabric.[6]

It was at this point, with the threat of demolition hanging over the buildings, that, in the standard medical histories, Lister came to save the hospital as the Victorians knew it. Whereas Simpson only had statistics to tackle 'hospitalism' and was able to offer the fundamental (but perhaps effective) solution of razing the buildings to the ground, Lister developed a much clearer theoretical insight into the nature of disease and was able to offer a rather less drastic treatment.

Joseph Lister

Joseph Lister was born in 1827, the son of Joseph Jackson Lister, a merchant, Quaker and keen amateur scientist (a Fellow of the Royal Society) who invented the compound achromatic lens for the microscope. Father and son were very close, and the son's interest in things microscopic was at least partly a conscious adoption of his father's mantle. Joseph Senior was a genial, lively, highly intelligent man with a wide range of interests. He was probably rather *more* intelligent than his son (he was certainly far wiser), but without the son's absolute concentration and dedication to a single area of research.

In 1845 Joseph Junior went to University College, London, then recently opened to enable non-conformists to obtain a university education. (Oxford and Cambridge insisted on students signing the 39 Articles of the Church of England.) Though intent on a medical career, he took a wide variety of courses in Greek, mathematics, botany and chemistry, as well as anatomy and physiology. Allied to what he had learned from his father, this gave him a far wider *scientific* grounding than the average medical men of his day. After obtaining his Bachelor of Arts degree, Lister concentrated on medicine and surgery, and became a dresser (a very junior assistant) to John Erichsen in 1851. In 1852 (there was so little medical knowledge then that it did not take long to qualify) he became a Bachelor of Medicine and a Fellow of the Royal College of Surgeons of England.

At this time Lister was advised by the Professor of Physiology at University College, William Sharpey, to pay a short visit to an old friend and colleague, James Syme, Professor of Clinical Surgery in Edinburgh, who was recognized as one of the cleverest surgeons in Europe. In fact, he stayed there for seven years and married Syme's daughter Agnes. Then in 1860 he was appointed Professor of Surgery at Glasgow University, and it was in Glasgow that he first developed antiseptic surgery.

He had early marked down 'hospitalism' – or, more scientificaliy, inflammation – to be his life's work. As a student he had written an essay on gangrene for a debating society and in 1856 he published a paper entitled 'The Early Stages of Inflammation'. Inflammation was an ideal field of medical research for someone with his background because it was of paramount medical importance and involved bringing microscopical techniques to bear on a surgical problem. As a further spur, his mother suffered from recurrent attacks of erysipelas.

Simpson had suggested that overcrowding, 'bad air' (it

was an old superstition that Black Death crept as a miasmal fog across the country) and dirt might be responsible for 'hospitalism'. Syme was convinced that wiping his hands on a clean towel before beginning an operation gave him better results. Lister in turn was of the school which tried 'cleanliness and cold water', that is, washing before operations to keep dirt away. This seems somewhat nonsensical, for if every wound is suppurating, if every bed is sodden, if all the bedclothes are filthy, why bother cleaning your hands? 'It seemed natural to postpone the cleansing of hands and instruments until the progress of dressings and probings had been finished' wrote one doctor.[7] Washing without knowing what to wash or why was doomed to failure and Lister achieved no improvement with this treatment.

Then, in 1865, he was given the single key idea that, right or wrong, enabled him to build a consistent framework on which to erect the edifice of antiseptic surgery. He was chatting about putrefaction with his friend, Thomas Anderson, Glasgow University's Professor of Chemistry, when Anderson suggested that he read the latest work of a French chemist, Louis Pasteur.

Pasteur proposed that tiny living organisms floating in the air and settling on organic matter caused its decay. Pasteur performed a classic experiment: he boiled broth in a glass vessel to kill any of these 'germs' it might contain and used the steam produced to drive out any residual air. On cooling, air was drawn back into the apparatus but had to pass through a long, convoluted glass spout which effectively filtered out all the grosser airborne particles. Thus only pure air re-entered the vessel. The broth it contained remained fresh. The same experiment was performed in an ordinary beaker open to the air and the broth soon 'turned'. So, suggested Pasteur, there were small living things, either free-floating or living on dust particles, which began to breed on entering the broth and caused its putrefaction.

Lister was struck by these papers: the putrefaction of broth and the putrefaction of a wound were not dissimilar; perhaps these small organisms caused suppuration. In one of his Ward Books (volumes of individual case notes kept on the patients in his wards by his house surgeons) there is an entry for 30 March 1865 for a Thomas Murdoch who had an operation on a

8

tubercular wrist. The operation was a success, but a month later Murdoch died:

> Latterly the wound took on a very languid action, approaching in character to Hospital Gangrene. In the next bed to patient lay a case of extensive lacerated wound of hand, which discharged freely, had an offensive odour and in the end took on Hospital Gangrene.[8]

Cases of 'hospitalism' such as this were instantly explicable on the germ theory: in a hospital there were lots of suppurating wounds as sources of germs to infect more patients. To confirm the hypothesis, Lister first checked Pasteur's experiments, using urine (which is naturally sterile) rather than broth, and blocked the germs' entry to his glassware with dry cotton wool. His experiments were successful and became prize exhibits, as Leeson recalled:

> Three flasks of aged urine, the most precious of the Professor's possessions, as sacred to him as the Three Hairs of Buddha are to the faithful Asiatic, he had had them for years, and he told me later, when he was appointed Professor of Surgery at King's College, of the concern and anxiety he had endured in transporting them to London, and how he and Mrs Lister carried them upon their knees all the way in a specially reserved first-class carriage to obviate as far as possible any evil that might befall them.[9]

Some of the flasks are still intact and have returned to Glasgow where they are preserved in the University's Hunterian Museum as a rather unlikely sort of holy relic, their contents rather darker than they were originally but still quite clear.

Surgical wounds, like broth, were *not* sterile, and Lister faced a rather more awkward problem than Pasteur, for he could hardly *boil* his patients! He needed some other way of killing germs. Over the years doctors had learned to apply a number of chemicals to wounds. They never understood why

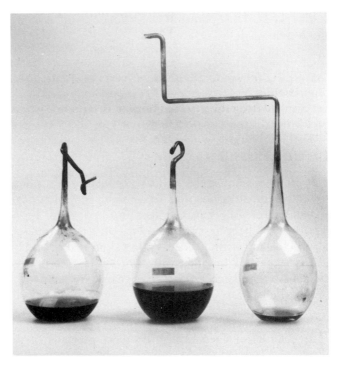

Flasks in which are preserved the still-clear samples of Lister's urine. (Hunterian Museum)

they did so except that occasionally, one presumes, these chemicals seemed to do some good. In Lister's own Ward Books are mentioned iodine, potassium permanganate, zinc chloride and potassium sulphite. All are disinfectants, though medical ignorance of their action can be gauged by the fact that doctors administered some of them internally. For cases of gangrene, fuming nitric acid – an extremely corrosive chemical – was used as a desperate last-ditch remedy. Medicine had thus inductively devised some ways of killing germs, but Lister's name will be forever associated with the addition of another disinfectant to the list: carbolic acid.

Lister read an anonymous newspaper article about some remarkable results achieved by the municipal sanitation department in Carlisle. By treating the municipal sewage with carbolic acid, they not only rendered the fields 'irrigated with the refuse material' odour free, but also killed off the bugs which usually infested the intestines of cattle pastured on those fields. The carbolic acid seemed to be killing off the germs responsible for the decomposition of sewage (producing the smell) and further annihilating the internal flora of these sewage-fed cattle, but *not* killing off the cattle themselves.

Through Anderson's good offices Lister obtained some carbolic to test its effects for himself. He convinced himself of its efficacy and started to use it regularly. But it was not the mere addition of another chemical to the medical arsenal that made the antiseptic revolution; the important factor was the development of a whole new method of applying carbolic acid, that is, the development of the antiseptic regimen, and this happened over a number of years.

The practice of antiseptic surgery grew out of a series of cases of compound fracture that Lister treated, and described in a classic paper published in *The Lancet* in March 1867 entitled 'On a New Method of treating Compound Fracture, Abscess, etc. with Observations on the Conditions of Suppuration'. Compound fracture was the ideal experimental test-bed for his ideas.

When there is a simple fracture – a clean internal break of the bone – its treatment, resetting and splinting are equally simple and also very effective. But in a compound fracture the break is so violent that broken ends of the bone are pushed out through the skin and a terrible wound results. At that time, as standards of hygiene at work and in the home were almost non-existent, such a wound almost always became infected. Amputation was usually the only remedy. In general, however, people with compound fractures were strong, healthy workmen with no other disease, and if infection could be kept at bay they should have recovered as well as simple fracture cases. Lister therefore had a goal to aim for, namely to make the treatment of compound fracture as safe as that for simple fracture. He had an obvious moral dilemma to overcome. If he amputated at the outset he would be able to save his patient's life 60 per cent of the time, at the going Glasgow rate. If his conservative treatment failed he could always amputate later, but by then it might be too late: suppuration might have set in too deeply, or might have so weakened his patient's constitution that further surgery became extremely dangerous. In the best Victorian paternalistic tradition Lister was prepared to run that risk.

His first case was Charles Cobb, admitted on 13 March 1865 with a compound fracture of the thigh. Lister's first attempt at an antiseptic treatment was to cover the wound with a piece of cotton soaked in carbolic and then splint the leg as usual. Already he had broken with tradition. By applying a disinfectant from the beginning of the treatment, even before surgery, Lister was preventing colonies of germs from becoming established, rather than hoping the wound would heal and applying the disinfectant only when suppuration was already present. Lister's own description of his treatment as *antiseptic* surgery, emphasizing the fight against sepsis with his new disinfectant, carbolic acid, is really rather misleading. What he was after, right from the beginning, was *aseptic* surgery, the prevention of germs from growing. Here, at his first attempt, Lister met with success, and by the middle of June Cobb was released with a sound leg.[10]

Lister was not so fortunate with his second case, Neil Kelly, who arrived just a week after Cobb, on 21 March. He also had a compound fracture of the thigh. Despite Lister's best efforts the wound turned septic 'in consequence, as I now believe, of improper management', as he sadly confessed in his *Lancet* paper. Lister was forced to amputate and did manage to arrest the spread of infection in time, since Kelly was discharged 'well' a year later (13 March 1866).[11] The fledgling antiseptic techniques were not adequate to keep a wound sterile.

On 12 August 1865 Lister's most celebrated case arrived. James Greenless, an 11-year-old boy (but already in full-time employment) was brought in with a compound fracture of the left leg, which occurred when he was run over by a cart. The wound was washed out with a solution of carbolic acid in linseed oil and then covered with 'carbolized' putty to keep it free from germs. Six weeks and two days later the boy was discharged with a sound leg. In his *Lancet* paper, Lister presented James G- as Case 1 in his epic sequence of successful applications of antiseptic treatment to compound fracture cases. Kelly was dismissed as an unsuccessful trial and so, to be scrupulously honest, Cobb also had to be ignored.*

As time went on, Lister developed and improved the treatment. The method of dressing changed, purer phenol (as we would now call the active ingredient in carbolic acid) was obtained and found to be soluble in water, so the linseed oil could be dispensed with. Weaker solutions were used to minimize the irritation caused to skin and flesh around the wounds. Different dressings were tried to hold the carbolic acid in place around the wound, and the 'spray' was introduced.

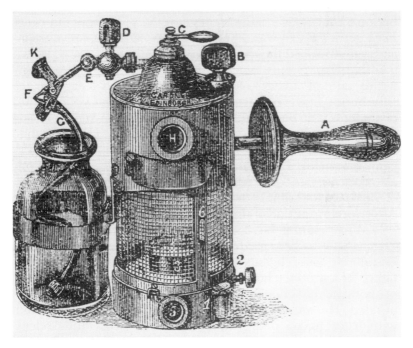

The steam spray. (Glasgow University Library)

---

* I am grateful to Dr Derek Dow, the Greater Glasgow Health Board Archivist, for drawing my attention to Cobb.

The spray was a sort of antiseptic anti-aircraft fire, intended to knock out any germs parachuting down in the direction of an open wound during surgery or while it was being dressed. A little boiler produced steam which atomized carbolic acid and wafted a fine phenolic mist over patient, surgeon and dressers. It was regarded as the ultimate weapon in the antiseptic surgeon's armoury.

In 1869 James Syme retired and Lister was appointed to succeed him in the Chair of Clinical Surgery at Edinburgh University. Few of the older generation of surgeons had been converted to his methods, since adopting the antiseptic regimen would have made their operations much more time-consuming because enormous attention was devoted to keeping out every *single* germ (or so it was thought). It was based on a revolutionary and unproved theory of the cause of disease: germs. Was it credible that Nature would act like 'some murderous hag?' wrote one of Lister's fellow surgeons from Glasgow. In Edinburgh, however, Lister gathered together his young guard of students who had graduated under his tuition and moulding or had read of his miraculous results and come to Edinburgh to receive the holy spirit at its fount. And thus antiseptic surgery came into being. Like many popular historical legends, this one also does not bear close scrutiny. It is a great oversimplification of the truth, and should be set against the picture painted in the Afterword at the end of this book.

What cannot be doubted is the reverence with which Lister came to be regarded in Victorian society. If antisepsis became a quasi-religious movement, Lister was a most unlikely figure for a prophet: he was aloof, shy, had a slight stammer and no political commonsense. He was, however, utterly single-minded. He was convinced that he had found the truth and, with true Quaker dedication, pursued its proof quite relentlessly in his lectures to students, in his operations and in the bacteriological research he carried out in his laboratory at home. If he had no conventional oratorical skills, his utter conviction and confessional honesty converted many. His personal magnetism comes across from almost every account. Even in an age much more self-confident than our own, his burning sense of purpose stood out.

William Henley and Margaret Mathewson

With postoperative infection kept in check, Lister was able to apply his antiseptic regimen to the whole of surgery and make full use of the freedom anaesthetics afforded. Perusal of his Surgical Ward Books reveals that the most common serious complaint he had to deal with, apart from compound fracture, was tuberculosis. His success here is far more difficult to judge. In the absence of a cure for the underlying disease, all he could do was to treat its local manifestations. He drained abscesses and was able to stop them becoming cross-infected most of the time, and he cut away carious bones and flesh. This left huge wounds which took months to heal, during which time they had to be prevented from turning septic. Furthermore, as patients suffering from tuberculosis had often been ill for a long time

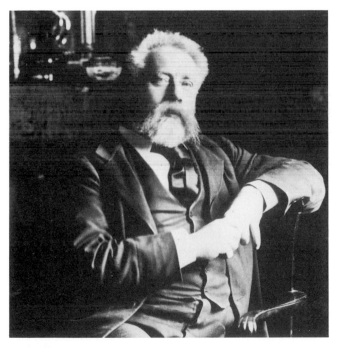

William Ernest Henley. (BBC Hulton Picture Library)

before coming to hospital, their general health had suffered and their natural resistance was low. And always the underlying infection remained, often to return later. None the less, Lister did achieve some remarkable results and patients started to come to him from all over the country.

One was William Ernest Henley, who was born in Gloucester on 23 August 1849. When he was 12 years old tuberculosis attacked the bones of his feet. His doctor's prescription was a visit to the slaughter-house, which was described by his brother:

> We both went next day. I was very sad, but he hopped along blithe and gay on his two crutches. An old woman who worked for my mother went with us. He and I both went into the slaughter-house, and saw a poor beast not long down and the butcher at work cutting open its inside. He greeted my brother with 'I'll be ready for 'ee in a jiff, Master Henley.' I was a bit scared, but my brother sat down on an old bench and I removed the covering of his bad foot. Then I saw the butcher drag a great mass from the beast's interior and pull it across the stone floor to where my brother was sitting, make a large slit in it with his big knife, and into this my brother put his bad foot, keeping it there for ever such a time, all the while talking to the butcher and his man in such a way that you would have thought he knew all about pigs, sheep and bullocks and their killing. [12]

His 'bad' foot had to be amputated, just below the knee, when he was 16.

His frequent illnesses (and his father's frequent near-bankruptcies) ruined Henley's education but, undaunted, he set out for London on his crutches intending to become a writer. This proved, as ever, a difficult task, and he was forced to live in considerable poverty in some of the less salubrious districts of the city. He was lucky to become friends with Harry Nichols, a genial and kindly man who ran a coffee house in the Commercial Road. Nichols plied Henley with warm food, warm whisky and warm friendship. He had, moreover, literary interests and encouraged Henley's ambitions.

Perhaps it was Henley's lifestyle (which he tried to

16

glamorize as 'Bohemian') that exacerbated his disease, for it now flared up again. He went to Margate to try the curative properties of sea bathing. His doctor, a Mr Treves, did not give him much hope. Henley wrote to Nichols:

> . . . I am afeared my marching days are over. *Exeat Bohemiensis!* . . . Indeed, my boy, my foot is powerful bad. Mr Treves tells me that if it suppurates, I shall have a devil of a turn with it. No more walking between tavern and tavern in the night – No more confabulations in the blue dawn: No more pipes in the winter evenings: no more pickles in the small hours! – Alas! and yet alas again! – An end is come to all these pleasant though highly improper things – My youth is dead. Knocked on the head at the early age of 23.[13]

In between these letters, which almost invariably end by begging for a small pecuniary donation, he wrote, read and tried to flirt with the maid, a Miss Crump.

Margate did his foot no good, nor seemingly much harm: 'It seems to stick in *status quo*', and Henley resigned himself to a long stay there. Then, rather suddenly, he decided to go to Edinburgh to see if Lister could save his foot.

Three biographies have been written about Henley. John Connell's (the third) is the most thorough and reliable, though he almost never mentions his sources. He writes that Henley read about Lister in the newspapers which 'had, of recent months, discussed freely and at length Lister's revolutionary methods, which old-fashioned practitioners denounced as charlatanry'.[14] (Why this should be happening in 1873, six years after Lister had first published his successful series of compound fracture cases, is difficult to tell.) The other two biographers, L. Cope Cornford and Kennedy Williamson, are generally less reliable, even though they both knew Henley personally. On this story they agree almost exactly word for word:

> . . . the surgeons at length told him that if his life was to be saved, the other foot also would have to come off. During

their parleys the doctors seem to have spoken scoffingly of Professor Joseph Lister (afterwards Lord Lister) who was then outraging the settled canons of medicine by his new-fangled antiseptic treatment. Henley made two retorts: with a stiff-jawed cussedness he avowed that his foot was not coming off, and that the man who was going to save it was Professor Lister.[15]

And so in August 1873 Henley set off for Edinburgh from London by sea, which was the cheapest way to travel about the country at that time.

Margaret Mathewson came to Lister from the island of Yell in Shetland. She was born in the parish school house at East Yell on 18 April 1848, the eleventh child of the parish teacher Andrew Dishington Mathewson, who was quite a remarkable man. In an almost illiterate society, his aunt taught him to read (the Bible, of course), write and to do some mathematics by the age of five. By the time he was six, local parents were bringing their children to *him* for lessons. Thus started on the road to pedagogy, he spent his whole life as a teacher on Yell where he taught full time until 1877, when he was 78. His classes catered for all ages from the five-year-olds up to young sailors, home for a season, who were revising trigonometry for their master's tickets. Even so, the fees he obtained as a teacher could not have kept his large family in a state of much luxury.[16]

Conditions were harsh in Shetland and most of the young people had to leave to find work. Margaret's brother Arthur was a shipping clerk in Granton, brother Walter worked for the lighthouse service and was currently in Campbeltown, and her third brother Laurence was in New Zealand. Margaret herself had probably been in service in Edinburgh.

Some time in 1874 she developed chest disease, the killer disease tuberculosis which was very common in the Highlands and Islands. In 1876 the disease moved to her upper arm and left her more or less incapacitated. In one letter she wrote: 'my arm is exceeding weak in itself, so much so that I cannot dress myself properly or haul the rug up in the night time; I can knit a little when it rests on my knee.' She was still determined to be a useful member of the family; indeed the family probably could not afford a passenger. At harvest time, in the autumn of 1876, she had had to help: 'One day going in the loft, the ladder slipped down among the peats and I fell across the loft door on

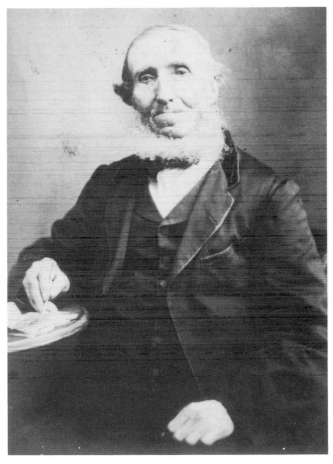

Andrew Dishington Mathewson. (Glasgow University Library)

my left side and my arm caught on a piece of wood. I thought it was broke quite snap as it sprang to the top of my head.' Where, as she puts it elsewhere, 'it had not been for 8 months previous.'

By the winter of 1876–7 things were becoming unbearable, and she decided to go to Edinburgh to see if surgery could help her. She faced a good deal of parental opposition to going, for her father knew full well what dangerous places hospitals had been. Margaret, however, had recently spent some time in Edinburgh and was aware that a change was occurring, as is clear from this letter she wrote to her brother Arthur on 31 January 1877, just before setting off on her eight-month ordeal:

> I may have to go to Edinburgh but cannot at present say when as the packet cannot get regular and there's such a bother lying in port for days together. I do not mean to say much about my half idea of going to Edinburgh as if I was telling them [it is not clear to whom this refers, perhaps some druggists in Aberdeen Margaret was consulting by post] or father etc. they seem to be so prejudiced against the name – Infirmary, doubtless only hearing about extreme cases – I have no such fears as I know girls who have gone there just to take a rest from service for a few weeks.

Certainly the best treatment that she could have been offered if she had stayed at home was gruesome. John T. Reid, who wrote a book entitled *Art Rambles in Shetland*, published in 1869, from which the picture of the interior of a typical Shetland cottage on p. x is taken, had this to say about contemporary Shetland remedies:

> A much-respected dissenting clergyman, still alive, called at this cottage to inquire for a poor woman who was dying of consumption. On hearing she was no better, he inquired if they had used means to aid her recovery: 'Yah,' said her aged mother, 'we gaed to the kirkyard, and brought *mould* frae the grave o' the last body buried, an' laid it on her breast. As this had nae effect, we gaed to the brig ower which the last corpses was tak'en, an' took some water frae the burn below, an' made her drink it. This failed too, an', as a last resource, we dug a muckle hole i' the grund, an' put her in't.'[17]

Opening pages of Margaret Mathewson's *Sketch*. (Glasgow University Library)

Mathewson and Henley represent the traditional poles of reaction to disease and death. They lived in an age when virtually no one achieved maturity without witnessing the death of some near friend or relative. Some 'accommodation' had to be made to death's imminent presence. Mathewson was a devout believer: she was not particularly worried about her earthly life because she was assured of an eternal spiritual life in heaven. If such an attitude seems remote today, even to believers, this is largely because medicine has removed death's threat for most of us until a comfortable old age. *Then* death was a much more personal enemy.

Henley was of the opposite school of thought. If death was ever present then concentrate on enjoying to the full the immediate moment, there might not be another. His concept of heaven was the warm whisky and friendship that Harry Nichols provided, to which he continually dreamed of adding a warm woman, but without much success. His attitude was, of course, also traditional. The backdrop of Boccaccio's *Decameron* is a group of wealthy young Florentines who, to while away a fortnight while the plague is raging all around, gather to enjoy food, sex and amusing stories.

ADMISSION

Margaret Mathewson   *Sketch*

Previous to my going to 'The Royal Infirmary', I knew I required an Introductory note; this is always given by the Rev. James Barclay, Minister of our Parish. I therefore wrote him, as I had resolved on going there for advice regarding my arm as it seemed to be getting worse.

Mr. Barclay kindly sent the note, also a box of ointment to dress the place he had previously operated on until I should get to Edinburgh. It was a rough passage all the way South, but I was not much sea-sick. There were no passengers I was acquaint with but one young gentleman from one of our villages, Daniel Scollay, Jnr, which was going out to Australia. He was indeed very kind and attentive. He had to go on to Glasgow and I to Leith, thus we parted at Leigh Walk station. I went to my friend Mrs. Barclay who was looking out for me. I then called on Cousin Martha and asked her if she would please accompany me to 'The Infirmary' and we went on Friday morning February 23rd. We came there at 10.30 a.m., met the porter at the gate and I asked him: 'If you please what's the best Professor's name for Surgery?'

'Professor Lister.'

'Thank you, please how will we find him?'

'Go down past that tree, then down stairs and to the lower house there facing you with two doors; go in the left hand door and up two flights of stairs; then ask for Professor Lister.'

'Thank you kindly.'

William Ernest Henley   *Letter to Harry Nichols,*
September 1873

I have passed through deep waters since I last wrote to you: here's the inventory. Wednesday, Aug. 20 – I set off from Wapping. Thursday 21 – I am somewhat seasick. Friday Aug. 22 – I land at Leith; train it to Edinburgh; cab it hither; arrive with exactly 10½ pence in my spleuchan (Scotch for purse idiot!); am informed by Mr. Lister that most probably my foot'll have to come off.

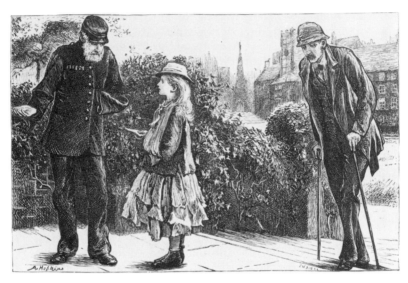

'The grey-haired soldier–porter bids me on'. Illustration from the *Cornhill Magazine* of 1875.

ENTER PATIENT in *Poems* (1898)

The morning mists still haunt the stony street;
The northern summer air is shrill and cold;
And lo, the Hospital, grey, quiet, old,
Where Life and Death like friendly chafferers meet.
Thro' the loud spaciousness and draughty gloom
A small, strange child – so agèd yet so young! –

Her little arm besplinted and beslung,
Precedes me gravely to the waiting-room.
I limp behind, my confidence all gone.
The grey-haired soldier—porter waves me on,
And on I crawl, and still my spirits fail:
A tragic meanness seems so to environ
These corridors and stairs of stone and iron,
Cold, naked, clean – half-workhouse and half-jail.

John Rudd Leeson   *Lister as I Knew Him*

He had about half of the old surgical hospital for his beds.
It was a grim, formal stone building of bastard classical
design, originally built for the old high school . . .

Smoke, dirt, and gloom surrounded his wards, which
facing east and west missed most of the little sunlight that
was available, and if the necessities of a modern entourage
are considered Lister had but a poor chance.

The buildings were old, their sanitary arrangements
primitive, and the wards neither lofty nor well lighted;
there were no through currents of air, the windows with
few exceptions being on one side of the ward, and those I
hardly ever remember opened. What outside air found its
way to the wards filtered in through dark and smelly
passages; the floors were sprinkled with sand, and though,
I suppose, they were occasionally washed I never saw
such process in evidence. But over and above all these
disadvantages the buildings had been infested for decades
with pyaemia and septicaemia, which still kept their
strangle-hold on the neighbouring wards of his colleagues.

The smell of the building was distinctive, a compound
of carbolic acid, stale tobacco smoke, and distant boiled
beef – the usual dinner of the patients. I have no reason to
think there were bathrooms as I never saw any.

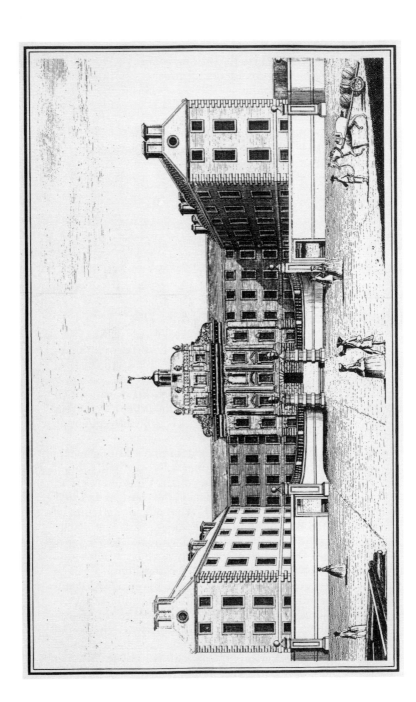

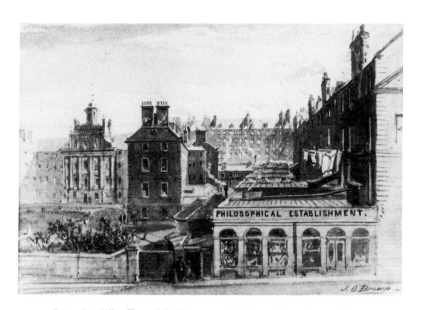

Opposite: The Royal Infirmary, Edinburgh as the architect dreamed it in 1738; *above:* The Royal Infirmary as it was in reality in the mid-nineteenth century. (Royal Infirmary, Edinburgh)

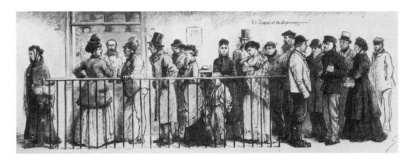

Queue of patients waiting for treatment. (BBC Hulton
Picture Library)

We passed on as directed and went up two stairs. On the
landing of the second we met Prof. Lister's House-
surgeon, Dr. Cheyne, a Shetland gentleman. I said 'Good
morning, sir, and can we see Professor Lister. If you
please.'

'You will see Prof. Lister in an hour or two, but what's
wrong with you?'

'A bad shoulder, sir.'

I then gave him Mr. Barclay's note, which in reading
the address, he seemed to know Mr. Barclay's write as he
instantly looked at me, then read it and then said, 'Do you
know me?'

'Yes, sir.'

'Who am I?'

'Dr. Cheyne – of Fetlar Shetland – sir.'

He then said 'Come this way into this room and I will
look at your shoulder.' And we went and he examined it.

'Were you thinking it out of joint?'

'Yes, sir.'

'No it is not out of joint. There's an abscess in the joint,
also another glandular abscess on the collar bone. You
will just put on only your outside jacket as Prof. will be in a
hurry when he comes and you will sit down on this seat
here in the lobby as our waiting room is made into a
bedroom at present, there being such a press of patients.'

'Thank you, sir.'

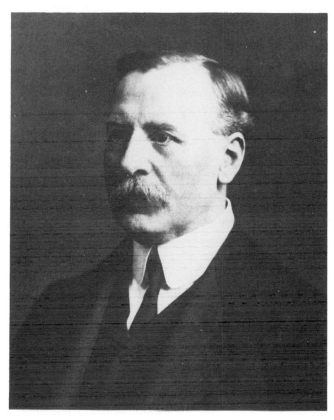

William Watson Cheyne. (By permission of the President
and Council of the Royal College of Surgeons of England)

William Ernest Henley

WAITING in *Cornhill Magazine* (1875)

A square, squat room that stinks of drugs and dust,
The walls and atmosphere a brownish drab.
The floor is foul; fair is the dressing-slab
With spotless lint, and tinware pure of rust.

A lank, bare bench shrinks round three sides and there
While certain smart young flippant Shallows tend
Such ills as Art incipient may amend,
Two endless hours I sit, and ache, and swear.

The decent woman strips her plastered eye;
The two old men their two old ulcers bare;
The boy, his leg unbandaged, starts to cry;

The girl, tight-lipped – 'Yon bluestane's awfu' sair!'*
To shut mine ears and raise my heart I try,
Thinking of darker hours that long since were.

Margaret Mathewson   *Sketch*

There was a lot of people with us, also waiting for advice.
While we were waiting there came upstairs an elderly
looking gentleman and next him Dr. Cheyne and then
quite a train of gentlemen behind. All went into a room on
the landing of the stair below us, but quite opposite where
we were sitting. They all took their seats as if it were in the
gallery of a church and in a little we heard fearful screams.
A little longer and all was quiet. Then we saw two students
rising up and they took a long basket (about six feet by
three) also sheets and pillows and made up a bed in this
basket. Then six or eight students came carrying a man
laid him in the basket, and carried him down stairs to the
ward. There were two women sitting at our side laughing
and talking. One of them said 'That's my husband that's
got his leg taken off. We will go now and there he's put.'

I said to Martha: 'That woman must be very cruel
hearted and I'm sure she is not worthy of a husband – to
sit here and carry on like that and her husband getting his
leg taken off.'

In a little there came a student out of the theatre carrying the man's leg rolled in silk paper and the blood tipping
from it, and went downstairs. It was indeed chilling to see

---

* Bluestone was crude copper sulphate used as an astringent.

it. Martha said, 'Dear-o-me! What a place to be in Maggie. I really can't stay long in here.'

'Well it does look to be a strange kind of work that's in this house, but doubtless it's a blessing there are some people who can do that sort of work.'

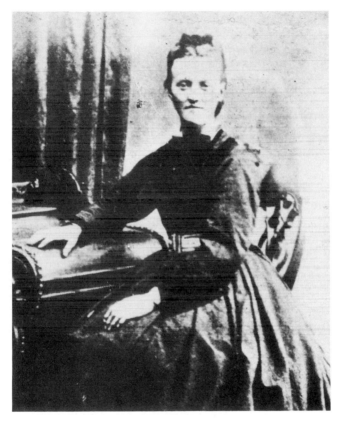

Margaret Mathewson. The date of the photograph is unknown, but she would appear already to have a diseased arm from the way she holds it. (Glasgow University Library)

Then a nurse came and told me to sit down next to the door, and put us all in the order we had arrived. In came Prof. Lister, Dr. Cheyne and a lot of students behind and all passed into the examination room. Dr. Cheyne called me in and introduced me to the Prof. as an acquaintance of his from Shetland. The Prof. examined the shoulder and asked:

'How did it first begin?'

'With a severe pain between the elbow joint and the shoulder joint, sir.'

'How long is that ago?'

'12 months, sir.'

'After it had continued between the joints some time did the pain go into the shoulder joint?'

'Yes, sir.'

'And always continued to increase.'

'Yes, sir.'

'Have you ever fallen on it?'

'Yes, sir, 4 months ago.'

'Where did you fall?'

'Going in a hayloft. The ladder slipt from my foot, sir.'

'And did anything strike this sore shoulder?'

'Yes, sir, a cleft of wood and made the arm go up to my head where it had not been for 8 months previous as it had been stiff in the joint.'

'Yes, just so.'

'What does this opening between the joints mean?'

'That is an operation the Rev. Mr. Barclay made a month ago, as it gathered there after I fell on it, sir.'

'How did a minister make the operation?'

'Because, sir, Mr. Barclay is all the practitioner that's in our island.'

There was at this time a chronic shortage of doctors in the Highlands and Islands of Scotland. The Royal College of Physicians of Edinburgh looked into the problem in 1852, and of 155 parishes investigated, 41 were rarely, if ever, visited by a doctor, and 52 were only 'partly' supplied with medical care. 'The college also found that in a number of places, Shetland in particular, the ministers and landowners still gave medical help.'

Such parishes, with a far-flung, poverty-stricken population, were obviously not financially attractive to the majority of doctors. With medicine then in a rather primitive state, it is not clear that this population was actually much worse off. That the local minister or landowner should dole out medicine was a long-standing tradition. Columba's monks used their medical skills as a weapon in converting the country; their medical mantle later fell on the educated, literate members of the community who could at least read herbals. Interestingly, in Yell, Margaret's island, in the eighteenth century it was the local blacksmith who seems to have looked after medical matters. He inoculated several thousand people against smallpox. [18]

In the Reverend James Barclay, Margaret Mathewson was more fortunate than most. His father had been a surgeon, on the neighbouring island of Unst, and so James no doubt acquired some medical knowledge. [19] Lister seems to have approved of his surgery but not of his physic.

Margaret Mathewson   *Sketch*

Prof. turned to Dr. Cheyne and said 'Is that correct Dr?'

'Yes, sir, she is saying quite true.'

'Well what do these marks mean that are all over your chest?'

'These marks, sir, are from a drawing plaster I had on some years ago.'

'What was that for?'

'For chest disease, sir.'

Professor then sat down, folded his hands, closed his eyes as if in silent prayer (which gave me more confidence in his skill). After sitting a little he rose up, came and felt it all over again, then took a silver probe about four inches long, probed with it through the open place on my arm. I felt the probe jagging in the shoulder cup. It was rather sore and bled a lot.

Prof. then asked, 'Have you ever had a cough?'

'Yes, sir, I had a severe cough and phlegm for about 3 months.'

'What did you apply for that?'

'Kays compound essence of linseed, chest powders, and cough plaster, sir.'

'All very good.'

'How long did you have chest disease?'

'For about 3 years, sir.'

'Have you any cough now?'

'No, sir.'

'Now, gentlemen, this quite accounts for the shoulder being diseased. The patient has had chest disease and has suffered a great deal from it but now instead of falling deeper into the lungs, it has Providentially turned from the lungs into the shoulder joint. Had not this operation been made on the arm it evidently would have returned to the lungs, and the patient would have died immediately, but this operation has drawn off a quantity of discharge. Well, we will sound your chest some day and see what we can do for you.'

'Thank you, sir.'

Dr. Cheyne helped me on with my jacket and made a sign for me to follow him. We went down stairs and into No. 3 ward.

Dr. Cheyne said, 'Go and take a seat at the fire and make yourself at home and the nurse will soon be here.'

'Thank you, sir.'

Martha was now beside us and she helped me to dress as I had been unable to dress myself for some months previously.

The right of admission to the Royal Infirmary lay solely with the surgeon and was made purely on medical grounds. There was no requirement, unlike the English Voluntary Hospitals, for a prospective patient to be interviewed by the Board of Governors. Nor were there any conditions on where a patient should come from: Henley arrived from Gloucester via London and Margate. On the other hand, certain parishes in Scotland contributed regularly to the running costs of the Infirmary: presumably in the last resort their residents received some sort of priority. Mid Yell was not one of these parishes, and so the note Margaret Mathewson felt she *required* from Reverend Barclay was not, strictly, necessary. But a note from a Minister confirming the details of a patient's complaint would never come in amiss.

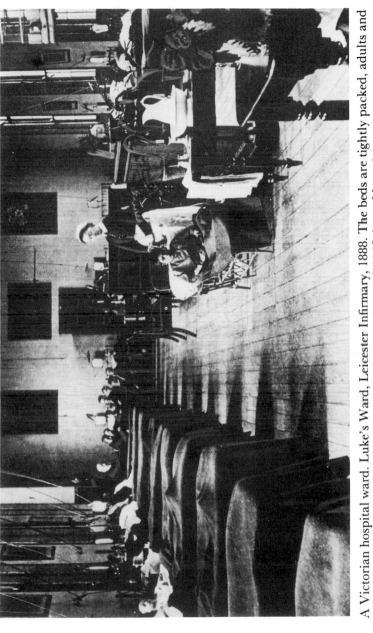

A Victorian hospital ward. Luke's Ward, Leicester Infirmary, 1888. The beds are tightly packed, adults and children share the same ward, and there is a bird cage (top right)! (*Leicester Mercury*)

In this case it would have been a heart-rendingly difficult decision for Lister to turn away a sick girl who had come all the way down from the Shetlands at her own expense to see him (especially since she was almost the neighbour of his house surgeon). Perhaps this is one reason why Lister's wards were always so overcrowded.

Henley's case is also interesting. He apparently had a sponsor: he had been recommended to Lister 'by a lady in the south of England . . . of very considerable influence in London society, and she has sent a pecuniary donation to the Infirmary.' The lady was apparently Lady Churchill and she had offered to pay Henley's hospital expenses, but Lister had replied that 'no expense would be incurred'.[20] There is no mention of Lady Churchill in the biographies of Henley, no evidence that he knew her (it is difficult to see how they would have met, or even, at that point, how she would have heard of him) and she certainly did not give *him* any pocket money during his stay.

Margaret Mathewson   *Sketch*

I then gave Martha £1 to give to Mrs. Barclay until I required it, and to tell Mrs. B. to wind my watch with her own until I see her. Martha said, 'Maggie, I'm real sorry to leave you here. Have you a nightdress with you?'

'Yes I put one in my satchel as I did not know but I might be kept in.'

'I will come soon back and see you.'

I went to the fire and sat down and took a look round. There were 9 beds and 8 patients in bed. All the beds had nice white covers on, clean pillow cases and clean sheets and the room so tidy and neat; also a big fire on. But I felt sad to see so many people in bed in one room, as I had never been in an hospital of any kind before. Under the beds was wood flooring. Down the centre was flagstone. On this stood a long table, on one end of which were lots of lotion bottles and dressing stuffs. On the walls were 8 pictures in frames and above the fire was a little bookcase full of books for our use, only 'Put it where you got it'; also the 'House Rules'. The walls were about 8 feet high and

4 air holes in the lathing like a church, 3 large windows. To the front below the windows were two drawers for our use and between the beds was a little high legged table for our meals and books. All the patients seemed to be quite at home and not to be suffering very much but no one spoke to me but all looking as if wondering if I was to be one of their number.

Being the first in the queue that day, Margaret was the first to be admitted. Later on more patients were sent down to No. 3:

Letter to her brother Arthur

No. 3 Surgical Ward,
Royal Infirmary.
Feby. 24th 1877.

Dear Brother Arthur,
    . . . There is 15 surgical patients in this ward and only 9 beds thus some beds has 3 occupants.
    I hear of no infectious disease i.e. I mean Small pox & Fever in the medical . . .

Margaret Cathn. Mathewson,
Professor Lister
No. 3 Surgical Ward
Royal Infirmary

In fact, overcrowding was a persistent problem in Lister's wards. He did not like turning away people he thought he could help. This meant patients sharing beds and/or extra mattresses being laid on the floor, as Margaret Mathewson notes elsewhere in her *Sketch*:

    . . . On Monday I was shifted to No. 1 Waiting Room where there were 2 beds only . . .
    I liked this little room much better than the big wards, as it was so quiet. There were more patients admitted and 2 beds had to be made up on the floor next day . . .

37

On Wednesday I again shifted to No. 3, and two patients got my bed in No. 1.

During this period, Lister was thinking of taking a Chair in London (see p. 133), and he felt obliged to clear up as many cases as possible before he went:

> ... there were so many patients at that time as Prof. Lister was intending to leave Edinburgh for London. There were 16 patients instead of 9 in No. 3. Thus we were upon the floor.

William Ernest Henley

THE WARD in *Cornhill Magazine* (1875)

Four long brown walls – a waste of plaster, bare
Save in some ragged prints; a glowing grate;
A flooring half of boards, half flagged with slate,
A crowd of bottles; space and light and air;

A lean gas pipe; a table slim and spare,
With bandages and lint; seven truckle beds,
Above whose coarse red rugs the horrent heads
Of seven pale poor devils turn and stare.

Some read; some knit; some sit up wearily,
Resting their arms upon their crooked knees;
Some sleep: more laughter comes from them, than moan.

This is a ward in hospital. You see
The field where Science battles with Disease,
And Hope – sweet Hope – succumbs to Death alone.

Just then, Miss Logan came in (our staff nurse). I rose up and said 'Good morning, ma'am.'

'Good morning, and are you going to be one of our number?'

'Yes, ma'am, for a short time I hope only.'

'Well, then we must treat you kindly. Just pull off your boots and make yourself at home as we are all very homely and social here.'

'Yes, ma'am, you seem to be that, and I would pull off my boots but I can't myself as I have got a sore arm.'

'Oh, then I'll help you.'

'Thank you ma'am but the nurse will likely be coming in soon.'

'Well, I am your nurse so just let me help you anyway I can.'

Miss Mary Logan was in charge of the Women's Ward and was one of a new breed of dedicated middle-class girls attracted into nursing by Florence Nightingale. In Edinburgh, the early 1870s were the watershed for nursing. In 1872 a Training School for Nurses was opened at the Infirmary to be run on Nightingale lines. A Miss Barclay, a Miss Bothwell and Angelique Lucille Pringle were sent up from St Thomas's Hospital, London to set it up. The following extract is taken from Miss Pringle's diary.[21]

Thursday Nov. 7th

Left St Thomas's at 9 a.m. the Matron seeing us off, also Miss Williams, Miss Airey and Miss Stains.

Had a most pleasant happy journey, a lovely day. Dined off Miss Nightingale's basket which was packed with all manner of good things.

November 8th, 9.30 a.m.

Went to the Infirmary, found our Lady Superintendent and Nurse Bothwell and had a nice reception and had got unpacked.

After a short stay went home and in the afternoon was
fetched by Miss Barclay. From this time am to remain at
the Infirmary. In the evening a message was brought from
the Matron Miss Forsyth that her assistant would be
ready at 7 to take Miss Barclay through the wards and
introduce her to the nurses. Miss Barclay agreed to this
and taking both of us with her set out punctually. First we
went to the ophthalmic wards which occupy the ground
floor of the wing.

A talkative smooth faced rather bonny woman received
us here. She spoke well of her under-nurse, Annie Fisher,
who worked about all day, and in the evening sleeps in the
female ward within call of the patients who are not
watched at night. Head nurse sleeps in a little room

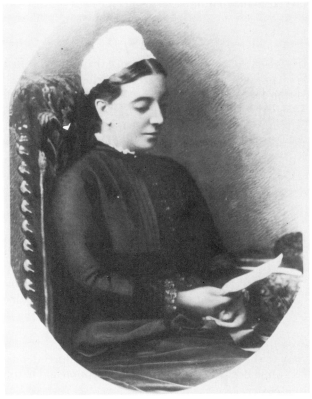

Miss Pringle. (Royal Infirmary, Edinburgh)

overhead with window into the ward. These wards were offensively close. They were neat but the scullery, etc., littered.

Leaving these we proceeded to visit the other wards. Most of the nurses received us kindly but there were some we could not help disliking. We found various night nurses about who had gone to bed at 12 returning at 5. They act in the threefold capacity of nightnurses, scrubber and assistant nurse.

One head nurse, Mrs. Porter, looked quite a dear old lady but her wards were not nice. She had been 27 years here and has now one of the heaviest charges.

Two of these day nurses were hideously deformed in face, quite unsuitable on that account alone for their post. Their wards looked nice however. The wards were all more or less close but none were otherwise offensive. There was no smell of wounds yet the closeness made one feel faint.

10th (November) Sunday
At 9 a.m. made a little round of the surgical wards. Found them only just beginning to work, nurses mostly very slovenly. Said they could not begin work till after breakfast which is served at light, so all is kept behind. The house surgeons visit at 10, the professors also visit on Sundays as they do every day of the week.

11th (November)
Nurse Bothwell went to wards 9 & 10 to get up the duties from Nurse Shaw who is leaving. Our nurse was impressed with the unwashed state of the patients and the slackness with which the diets were drawn. She observed that the night nurses did all the ward work, the surgeons all the dressings, the day nurse spending most of her time in her own room.

17th (November)
A great many night nurses still lingering about at work though it was past 5 and they had to return at 11. Wondered how they stood it.

Tea at 6. Then went to bed with Miss Barclay. Tried very hard to sleep but could not. Talked instead and got so beautifully warm for the first time since arriving in

Edinburgh that we were not positively glad to be called at 11. Got up however, dressed, had supper and at midnight went to the wards. Eye wards first. Both dark, several patients awake, no nurse visible in bed or out of it. Kitchen in a blaze of light, very dirty, fire out, frying pan among the ashes. Empty glass on the table and under it poor old Annie Fisher, dead asleep. After many failures, we succeeded in rousing her sufficiently to speak. She lay still quite at her ease, very good natured, and without the least apprehension of the circumstances made us some random answers.

Miss Barclay said: 'What about your patients, Nurse?' She answered with a laugh, 'Oh, I had nae mind o'them' which we thought a (?) skilful epitome of the state of nursing. We raised the day nurse and made her come down and take charge. She insisted that the woman was overtired but not drunk. Leaving them we went on to the other wards, going right over the hospital.

We found several nurses asleep in bed, in some instances in the male wards. Those who were awake were mostly sitting over the fire wrapped in a blanket, already heavy with sleep. These were very pale all of them, some were sodden, some were stupid old women, some slovenly young ones of the lowest class. Early in the round we were followed up by old Annie Fisher, furiously enraged, screaming insolence at us. She 'had seen a good many out and she would see us out too.'

18th (November) 2.30 a.m.
Began a round of the wards. With few exceptions they were lighted up and the nurse was scrubbing. It is an institution here that the wards shall be scrubbed every Monday morning beginning at 2 o'clock. Therefore on this round we found none asleep though we saw that some had been by the arrangements near the fire. Very many of the patients were awake, through the scrubbing and those who were ill were in no instance receiving attention.

In the forenoon Miss Barclay gave notice to the night nurse of No. 7 Surgical to leave (Maria Campbell) having a bad report of her from the day nurse and from her own observation, considering her quite unsuitable. The woman, who had a rough appearance and surly manner threatened to go to the doctor who had recommended her. Miss Barclay went to Miss Forsyth to enquire about this recommendation and heard the following story. As a very young girl Maria Campbell was left friendless in exposed circumstances. To protect herself she assumed male clothing, which she continued to wear for fifteen years without detection supporting herself during that time as a navvy. About a year ago being seized with smallpox her sex was discovered and Dr. Littlejohn on her recovery being anxious to help her and able to recommend her as strong, sober and honest, sent her to the Matron of the Infirmary. Miss Forsyth put her on duty as a night nurse on trial till the new Lady Superintendent should come. Miss Barclay does not think the history at all a sufficient reason for keeping her on as a nurse, but will try to employ her as a scrubber.

19th (November)
Found much comfort in going and coming in the wards today. The patients get to look out for us and are pleased to see us, and some of the nurses look friendly. In the evening Mr. Renton, Dr. Watson's house surgeon brought

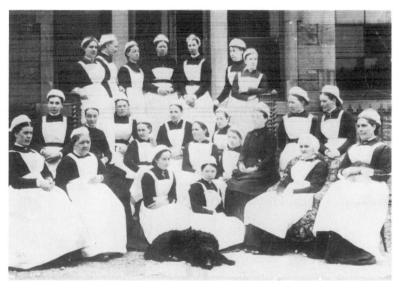

A group of Nightingales, the new style of nurses trained in Florence Nightingale's precepts. (Royal Infirmary, Edinburgh)

43

some gentlemen through our wards 9 and 10 to show them the improvement already wrought.

21st (November)
At half past eleven o'clock Miss Barclay and I started on a round of the wards.

We found in nearly all the gas blazing the day nurses running about and a perfect riot of laughing and talking going on among the nurses and patients. Nurse Porter's wards were the noisiest, the old lady herself being very loud. Into one ward which at first we found quiet, though without a nurse, and in which there was at least one patient in a most critical state, two of the nurses rushed in the noisiest manner startling the poor fellow shockingly.

Our own wards presented a pleasing contrast and we appreciated more than ever before what had been attained at St. Thomas's in the way of system. The gas was lowered, the patients asleep, the night nurse long ago quietly in charge.

And so, smoothly and (mostly) calmly, the Nightingale nursing revolution took place.

Although Miss Logan was in charge of the Women's Ward and would not under normal circumstances have had anything to do with Henley, at one stage he shared a room with two boys, Roden Shields and William Morrison, and she took especial care of them outside her normal duties. Through her visits to the children, Henley got to know her.

William Ernest Henley

STAFF-NURSE: NEW STYLE in *Cornhill Magazine* (1875)

Blue-eyed and bright of face, but waning fast
Into the sere of virginal decay,
I view her as she enters, day by day,
As a sweet sunset almost overpast.

44

Kindly and calm, patrician to the last,
Superbly falls the gown of sober grey,
And on her chignon's elegant array
A cap receives the impress of her caste.

She talks Beethoven, frowns disapprobation
At Balzac's name, and sighs at Madame Sand's,
Knows that she has exceeding pretty hands.

Speaks Latin words with due accentuation,
And gives at need, as one who understands,
A draught, a judgement, or an exhortation.

A different view of Miss Logan from that of Henley is provided by Roden Shields. He later wrote of her that 'she was the daughter of an Auld Licht minister,* who had reared her piously, educated her liberally, and, dying, left her unprovided for materially.' Shields described her as 'a broad-minded, cultured Scottish gentlewoman', and continued:

Henley does her scant justice; he could not know her as I did. For over two years she was my foster-mother rather than a professional nurse. Although outside her proper duties, she used to bath me regularly, personally see to my food and medicine, and frequently carry me to her sitting-room for a change and to play with her collie. Again, on a rare occasion she would hire a carriage and take me for a two hours' drive, my garb on such emergencies being a half-blanket, a shepherd's tartan plaid, and a Glengarry bonnet. I remember the hysterical dry sob that would rise in my throat as we bowled along Princes Street, Miss Logan in a hackney carriage, but I in a chariot of fire rushing through Wonderland, wheels whirling in my brain, fresh air and bright sunshine bewildering me;

---

* During the eighteenth and nineteenth centuries, the complex relationship between Church and State caused the Church of Scotland to break up into different sects at an alarming and utterly confusing rate. The 'Old Lights' split (over the status of the Covenant) from the Burghers who had split (over the Burgess oath) from the Seceders who had split (over patronage) from the Church of Scotland.

feeling as a child only could feel who had been long immured in hospital.

On other occasions she would carry me off to tea with Mrs. Porter or some other of the staff-nurses or under-matrons.

I often think I should have died had Miss Logan confined her attentions to me within the limits of her professional duties; but her love and sympathy continued when duty left off. She has spent her life doing what she could (which was a great deal) for the stricken ones among whom her lot was cast.[22]

Although the Nightingales had arrived, there were plenty of the old school still around. The most celebrated of these was

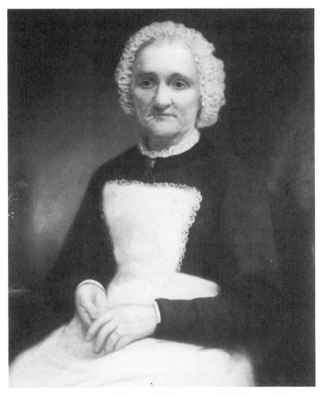

Mrs Porter. (Royal Infirmary, Edinburgh)

Mrs Porter who, though crusty, was exceptional in that she *was* a dedicated nurse. She had served under Syme and by then had become part of the hospital folklore:

The presiding genius of the wards was Mrs. Porter. I beg her pardon, I ought to have said Mistress Porter, as this was how she was addressed in accordance with the national etiquette of her class.

She must have been well over seventy. Her hair was white, her face lined and wrinkled, but her complexion would have done credit to a girl in her teens. Her eyes were of a cold piercing blue, searchlights, but could at times twinkle with a roguish humour, conveying both instruction and rebuke. She wore the tightly laced corsets of the period which, struggling with a protuberant abdomen, lifted her waist almost to her arm-pits: her snow-white, closely fitting, goffered cap, and capacious white apron, showed to advantage against her grey-blue stuff dress, which looked as though it had never been new or would ever get old. She had long lost her teeth, and would have considered artificial ones a reflection upon the arrangements of the Deity, and would munch her jaws with significance when rouses or angered.[23]

Everyone delighted in adding to her reputation.

One sees again the worthy nurse, Mrs. Porter, making her nightly round, candlestick in hand, towel over arm, bearing a tray of requirements, as she called, 'Wha' says ile, wha' says peels?'*

Her Lister worship was intense, yet she would attempt her authority, dog his footsteps and, as he approached the stairhead on his way to the wards downstairs, would gently filch the towel from his hand saying, 'Excuse me, Mr. Lister, but gin' my towels gang doon below, they ne'er come up again.' Thorough and good-hearted, many

---

* I think this means, approximately, 'Who'd like beer, and who'd like lemonade?'

were the kindnesses she showed to poor patients who
would find, on the morning of their discharge, small sums
of money under their candlesticks to help them on their
way home.

The tears ran down her cheeks when Lister went to
London. In later years, in her little room which was
tapestried with photographs of former residents and
others, she found herself ever surrounded by old friends,
and as she indicated her air cushion would say, 'An, I'm
sitting on Dr. Ronaldson.' She would sigh as she remarked,
'We've nae Listers or Symes noo, but we try our little
best.'[24]

Henley wrote a poem about her, picking up this hospital
legend.

STAFF-NURSE: OLD STYLE in *Poems* (1898)

The greater masters of the commonplace,
Rembrandt and good Sir Walter – only these
Could paint her all to you: experienced ease
And antique liveliness and ponderous grace;
The sweet old roses of her sunken face;
The depth and malice of her sly, grey eyes;
The broad Scots tongue that flatters, scolds, defies,
The thick Scots wit that fells you like a mace.

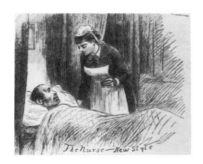 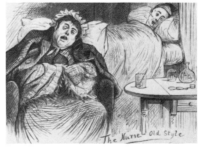

The nurse, new style and old style. (BBC Hulton Picture
Library)

48

These thirty years has she been nursing here,
Some of them under Syme, her hero still,
Much is she worth, and even more is made of her.
Patients and students hold her very dear.
The doctors love her, tease her, use her skill.
They say 'The Chief' himself is half-afraid of her.

Margaret Mathewson   *Sketch*

Then the dinner bell rung, and the nurse came in with
9 basins of soup and bread on a tray. Then she came back
with potatoes and meat. At 4.30 p.m. the tea bell rung and
nurse McConnachy again came with tea, bread, and
butter.

At 5 p.m. visitors came and stayed till 6.30 p.m. when a
bell rung for them to leave. At 7.30 supper came, bread
and milk. At 8 p.m. all had to go to bed that were walking
about. 8.30 a change of nurses — the day nurses went off
duty and the night nurses came on. I lay awake about
1½ hours then went asleep.

Next morning I was awoke by the night nurse (Michi)
at 5.30 a.m. 'Get up and make yourself generally useful.'

'Oh yes, I am willing to give you my one hand.'

'Where have you put the other?'

'Its here yet but next to useless.'

'Well I hope it will soon get well if you stay with us any
time.'

For breakfast we first for a basin of porridge and milk,
then coffee and bread. About 9 a.m. there was a change of
nurses again also the morning post called with letters for
the ward. At 9.30 a.m. Miss Logan came on duty. At 10
she came with an armful of gauze 40 yds to the patients to
tear into lengths of 20 yds each, some about 3 inches wide
and others less for bandages. These were smoothed, then
rolled on a little hand machine for the purpose, then put
into a little basket and set on the table with other dressings
stuffs.*

---

* Lister was notoriously profligate in his use of bandages (see p. 86).

49

10.30 people began to call to see Prof. Lister. 11 and 11.30 there was a great commotion. Doctors driving in to the door, students by scores walking down from the college arm in arm. Then the two surgical Professors came each in his own open carriage, viz. Prof. Spence and Prof. Lister. At 11.40 a.m. all was very quiet. 12.45, Prof. Lister, Dr. Cheyne and about 40 students came downstairs, and into our ward, examined some of the patients, then came to me and the Prof. said 'Undress please.' I did so very reluctantly but Miss Logan came and helped me so as not to detain the Prof. The Prof. then asked me almost the same questions as on the previous day, then said to the students 'Gentlemen, this is a case of consumption of the lungs but is providentially turned from the lungs to the shoulder joint. There it has formed a circumficial abscess. Also here is another glandular abscess on the collar bone which makes this a very interesting case for us all. Dr. you will dress it antiseptically this afternoon.'

They all went out. The Doctor came and dressed it with carbolic lotion and it felt much easier.

At 1 p.m. all the students had to return to the college, but Prof. always had some operations to perform before he left. Then the dressers (students who had to put in 6 months at dressing cases in 'The Surgical' then 6 months in 'The Medical' ere they can graduate) came and dressed both out and indoor patients, and often those outdoor patients had very disagreeable sores.

John Rudd Leeson   *Lister as I Knew Him*

Lister's staff consisted of twelve dressers, three clerks, and a resident surgeon (or as would more generally be called, house surgeon). The appointments were for six months, and personal application was necessary.

It was generally the best men who applied for the dresserships; those who had done well in the classes and were interested in their work, as they knew they would get little examinational help from him and would be led into paths that were outside the curriculum, as no examiner would then have dreamt of officially recognising anti-septics, much less of making them a test. The curriculum was crowded, and the examinations pressed closely upon each other, and it required both courage and enthusiasm to spend valuable time upon that which had no marketable value.

Lister's dressers were largely serving-men. They held tins of lotion, fetched and carried, and lifted and moved the patients; but were never allowed to dress serious cases. They were learning antiseptics and struggling for a clerk-ship later on, and as only three clerks would be chosen out of the twelve dressers the competition was severe.

To Lister, his dressers were always 'Mr.'; he never called us by our surnames only. No matter what the emergency, this epithet was never omitted. We did not quite like it; we did not actually dislike it, but we felt it was a little barrier. He invariably treated us with the most courteous regard, as indeed he did every one, but habitual politeness is rather embarrassing; he was shy and we were restrained.

The clerks were the non-commissioned officers of the squad, and did responsible work; in addition to which they instructed and superintended the dressers.

I was never more surprised than when, on the last day of the course, my name was read out a medallist; of course, I knew it meant a clerkship.

The clerk's work was apportioned, one for the spray, one for the instruments, and one for the chloroform, each in rotation for two months. They had to take notes of the cases, and dress them as soon as the risk of operation contamination was past. Four dressers were assigned to each clerk, who had to break them in, teach them their minor duties, and initiate them into the mysteries of the antiseptic ritual; it was responsible work, and we were sensible of our trust.

Antiseptics were on their trial and had to win their spurs, and if through our fault a case went wrong, which I am pleased to say it seldom did, the eyes of the foreigners were upon it and the truth of Lister's theories was at stake.

One afternoon I was dressing a case of psoas abscess, and the Professor made a surprise visit, accompanied by two foreign professors. They paused at the foot of the bed, Lister explaining the case and expounding the dressings,

and then in a most impressive voice, said: 'If this gentleman dares to let a single germ enter this wound he will be
as culpable as though he took his scalpel and plunged it
into the patient's carotid.'* The foreigners bowed in polite
acquiescence, and glared at me as though I were some
dangerous animal. To my relief they soon passed on, and
instinctively I dipped my hands in carbolic lotion and
hoped I had not betrayed my trust. It was no light matter
working under such responsibility, but this was the spirit
in which all the work was done; we knew that Lister relied
upon us not to fail him.

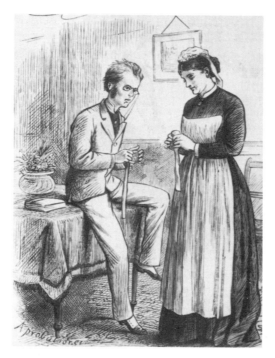

A young doctor learning his art. (BBC Hulton Picture
Library)

---

* Lister erroneously thought that abscesses were sterile until they had been
opened.

Over the clerks and dressers was the resident surgeon (house surgeon), who was a graduate, and had charge of the wards in the Professor's absence; he was a busy man and rarely off duty. He held the appointment for six months and was chosen from the clerks.

The Professor paid his daily visit at noon. For half an hour before, a general bustle ensued, above which the hissing of the sprays was heard getting up their steam. The head nurse, Mrs. Porter, was now in evidence, giving her orders right and left, clearing the course, and seeing that everything was in readiness; moving rapidly from ward to ward, desperately in earnest. Slowly and solemnly the open landau and pair of horses turned the corner at the top of the hill, and carefully descended to the hospital yard; we knew its clatter as it rumbled over the stones. It was a dignified equipage and Lister looked well in it, looked the part every inch. The crowd of students was gathering, generally some thirty or so, and the foreigners were turning up. The Professor quickly alighted, and though well over fifty and inclined to stoutness, tripped up the stairs often taking two at a time, to the upper floor where was his private room. They say that great men never run – Aristotle in his Ethics goes further and says: 'The high-minded man will be slow in his movements;' but Lister hurried to his work, and even in passing from ward to ward walked briskly. Arrived at his little room, hardly more than a few feet square, he was closeted for a few minutes with the house surgeon, and then a reception of the visitors was held. They were a grotesque collection of Scandinavians, Danes, Germans, Russians, Poles, French, Italians, Americans, and Japanese, rarely less than two, and generally three or four. There was a great deal of bowing and card presenting, Lister most graciously receiving them all, smiling kindly, and inquiring now in French, and now in German, about his foreign friends who had given them their introductions. After a few minutes a start was made for the wards (Mistress Porter had now retired to her little room and was earnestly knitting, apparently unconscious that anything was going on!), Lister dividing his attention between the foreigners and the leadings of the house surgeon. He spoke French and German fairly well, and the foreigners seemed to understand, or were too polite to show they didn't.

53

They were a strange medley: the distinctive cut of their clothes, the shortness of their hair, the heaviness of their moustaches, the diversities of their noses, and their invariable myopia, nearly all of them wearing glasses, unusual to Britishers of that day.

A bed approached, the patient was greeted with the kindly smile, and the dressing examined to see whether the discharge had 'come through', and if it had, a change of dressing was imperative.

A change of dressing being required, the spray was turned on and basins of 1 in 40 carbolic lotion handed, into one of which scissors, forceps, probes, and instruments were cast, whilst the hands of the workers were immersed in another. Lister insisted upon having a piece of gauze always put into the lotion for washing purposes, and it is strange how often this was forgotten – there are some things which seem doomed to be forgotten! Time after time he would turn to the dresser, and plaintively ask, 'How can I apply the lotion with my fingers?' The bandages were then cut with bulb-pointed scissors to avoid pricking the patient, and the corner of the dressing carefully lifted, particular care being taken that a full cloud of spray followed the dressing as it was being removed; the Professor then smelt it, and then carefully smelt all round the edges, and after a smile of satisfaction that it was 'quite sweet', would hand it round to the foreigners to verify the fact.

When all was finished he would say to the patient: 'Now are you quite comfortable?'

Margaret Mathewson   *Sketch*

Post came again at 3.30 p.m. visitors at 5 p.m.; supper at 7.30 and read a chapter, then prayer which closed the day much better.

I soon went asleep but awoke about 11.45 and was thinking on what I had seen and heard these 2 days some of which I thought very strange. While thinking thus, the door opened and Dr. Cheyne came in and went to each patient and seemed to be looking what position they slept in. He came to me.

'Dear-o-me! how are you awake at this time, 12 o'clock?'

'I awoke a little, ago, sir.'

'Have you any pain in the arm?'

'Not at present, sir.'

'Do you feel much pain in it when about going asleep?'

'Very much at times, sir, and often it wakens me out of sleep.'

'Just so; Oh well, I hope you will get free of all your pain ere you leave us, and Good night.'

'Goodnight, sir.'

Next morning was Sunday. Things went on as usual until 9 a.m. A change of nurses and all was quiet. I took a book and sat down and read a piece, then thought I shall try and read a piece to some of these people. Just then the door opens and one of the dressers a Mr. Abercrombie came in with the Bible and Hymn book in his hand and gave out the hymn 'The great physician'. He then read the first part of the 12th Chapter of Matthew, dwelt most on the man with the 'withered hand', spoke of what great difficulties the man must have experienced for want of its use, then how miraculously it was restored, then Christ's healing power and how he still retains the same power to the present moment and is the Physician of the soul as well as the body.

I enjoyed this meeting very much indeed. At 10.30 a.m. people came for advice as usual (to my surprise) and all went on as usual, and I was told that the most serious operations were generally reserved for Sunday. We had tea ½ an hour earlier, and the visitors gate was opened at 4 p.m. instead of 5 p.m. and I had 4 friends among them. Their company for 2 hours cheered me up a little, but I felt sorry to see them go away without me, and I had to be shut up with strangers inside of those huge walls and folding gates. However, though it does look bleak and dreary yet it is a hospital and not a prison and I am here for no crime only under the wise dispensation of my heavenly Father and He will do with me just as he sees best.

The city of Edinburgh closed down on a Sunday in that highly religious era. Lister himself, when Syme's house surgeon, had once failed to keep the Sabbath properly, and been duly punished for it. He had been led onto Arthur's Seat, the volcanic cliffs that give Edinburgh such a spectacular back drop, by John Beddoe, a fellow doctor and experienced mountaineer:

> I suppose much experience of the place had made me careless. A large fragment came away in my hands, and the stone and I both fell upon Lister. He was looking up at the time, and squeezed himself cleverly against the face of the cliff; but the huge stone struck him on the thigh with a grazing blow, and then whirled down the talus below with leaps and bounds, and passed harmless through the middle of a group of children who were playing hopscotch at the bottom right in its way.
>
> Lister was badly bruised, but no bone was broken. I went off at once to the Infirmary and procured a litter and four men, wherewith I returned to Lister. As our melancholy procession entered the courtyard of the surgical hospital, there met us Mrs. Porter, the head nurse then and for many years after. She wept and wrung her hands, for Lister was a universal favourite.
>
> 'Eh, Doketur Bedie! Doketur Bedie! A kent weel hoo it wad be. Ye Englishmen are aye sae fulish, gaeing aboot fustlin upo' Sawbath.'
>
> I do not suppose Lister ever whistled on Sunday. I am certain I did not . . . but we had suffered from the national offence. We were both in bed for a fortnight . . .[25]

THE OPERATION

Margaret Mathewson   *Letter of 6 March 1877 to her father*

. . . There was a woman carried in on a board with a bruised thigh bone and put in my bed so I have got another bed in a nice little room where there's only one bed besides occupied by another old woman whose arm is taken off at the shoulder. She suffers a great deal with it . . .

Sketch

On Monday I was shifted to No. 1 Waiting room where were 2 beds only. One of them was occupied by an old woman, looking very ill, also dejected and anxious.

'What is wrong with you?'

She held up her left arm, which has been amputated to an inch above the elbow.

'What was wrong with it ere it was taken off?'

'It was burned and never got better but got blue and bruised like.' (That means putrid.)

After some conversation with her I went to bed, but had not slept long until I was awoke by her moans of pain and wailing lament. I got up and asked her if I could do anything. She said 'It's the pain, the pain.'

'Have you no pillow below your arm?'

'No.'

'Well hold it up and I'll put one of mine below and it will feel easier I think.'

She then said, 'It is surely the Lord that's sent you to me.'

'Well perhaps he is.'

I then spoke to her on religion a little, but I saw she was quite a stranger to that, and I am sorry to say as far as I know she remained so.

On Wednesday I got some letters from home which cheered me up a little. Thursday, there were some patients sent to the Convalescent and others admitted, and I again shifted to No. 3, and two patients got my bed in No. 1. Granny cried when she knew I was to be shifted. I always went and cheered her up, but I had got the idea that I would lose my arm assuredly as she had lost hers.

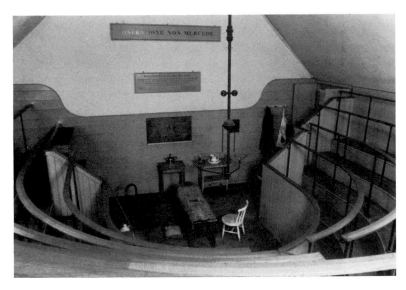

A Victorian operating theatre.

Next day I was called upstairs to be lectured on, and was put into a dark room where I found by their voices there were others before me. There were 2 doors in this room and a porter at the front one to let out any who were called into 'The Theatre'. This dark room was called 'The amphi-theatre' but oftener it was called 'The dark hole'. I sat about 2 hours and then Dr. Cheyne came and told me I was not wanted today as there were so many others.

'Thank you, sir.'

The next day nurse came in the waiting room (No. 1) to me and said 'Maggie, you are to undress and be ready for upstairs and here's a blanket to put round you so as not to take cold sitting in the dark hole so many hours perhaps.'

I did so and sat down and in a little Dr. Henly (a German Dr.) came and called me upstairs.

I sat two hours in the dark hole again. Then Dr. Cheyne came and told me I was not wanted today yet as there were so many to be done. I was truly glad as I was shaking with fear and cold as well. When I came downstairs I found I had lost my dinner but I went and got a piece. Next day I was called again, and was also called into the big theatre and lectured on before about 40 gentlemen and all the lecture was in English so I had the benefit of it too. Prof. asked me almost the same questions (as there were some gentlemen present who were not the previous days) as he had done previously; then again explained the case as before, thus

'Gentlemen this is a very singular case of consumption of the lungs, both being a little affected, but it has very Providentially taken a turn and gone off the lungs and seated in the shoulder joint, there forming a circumficial abscess. Also here's another glandular abscess near the collar bone. The patient must have been no stranger to suffering as you see here the form of the chest bones, also the singular shape of the shoulder joint.'

I was very much excited by this time, so much so that I felt the cold perspiration running down my forehead which the Prof. observed then patting me on the arm said: 'Now turn your back on these gentlemen.'

I was thankful to hear this but on turning round my feelings were more aroused by looking on the blackboard and seeing the diagram of my arm chalked in its then swelled state, also the natural state, then special marks where it had to be operated on. Seeing this I almost fainted as until then, I had a hope it would not be so serious an operation. Dr. Cheyne came and took my arm and helped me downstairs and told the nurse to put me to bed and stay with me a little. I lay down for about half an hour and then got up and went out, for the fresh air (that is such fresh air as is there but it can't bear the name of fresh air).

I had a short walk and felt much better, then returned to get a piece but the nurse had got strict orders to give me

59

none until teatime as I was to be done tomorrow and the stomach had to be as empty as possible for the vomiting which generally follows chloroform. Ere teatime I felt rather hungry, having had nothing from 8.30 a.m.

Margaret's first-hand account rather destroys the following standard hagiographical passage of Leeson.

John Rudd Leeson   *Lister as I Knew Him*

The theatre was a large, lofty, square apartment, bald and formal, lighted by a large window on the north side.

A large blackboard filled the space under the window, and on this Lister would draw. He was not a skilful draftsman, but his diagrams were to the point and helped us to understand the matter.

The method of clinical teaching was distinctive and unusual; it consisted in bringing the patients from the ward into the theatre, where the students were conveniently seated for seeing and taking notes.

One would have thought it would have been too trying an ordeal for a patient to find himself suddenly confronted with six hundred eyes, but they seemed to like it; they were never resentful and rarely seemed nervous. On the contrary, they appeared to appreciate the attention they were receiving, and that so many 'doctors' were interested in and concerned with their case.

The patient was brought in by the dressers; there were never any nurses in the theatres much less a 'theatre sister'. They underwent no special treatment, neither washing nor scrubbing of the part, and were clad in their ordinary garments; the severer cases were carried on a stretcher by the dressers.

They were invariably greeted by the Professor with his sweet and assuring smile; he would hand them to a chair or assist them to get on to the table. The magic of that smile allayed all fear, and in its sunshine they felt the moment of their deliverance was near; his presence and kindly attention filled them with comfort and hope, and they knew that all that was humanly possible would be done for them.

A description of the case followed and its special points were elucidated; then one or two of the distinguished foreigners who were generally present were invited to examine the part. Every stage of the investigation was conducted with the utmost regard for the patient's feelings: technical terms only were used, and nothing was said or suggested that could in any way cause them anxiety or alarm.

He had no natural gift of expression, and I am sure disliked public speaking and was haunted by the dread of the little stammer which never left him. His words were carefully chosen and deliberately uttered, and he rarely failed to make his point; he carried us along with him, and perhaps no teacher was ever better remembered. It was his earnestness that was his eloquence, and his concern for the patient his motive power.

These lectures were very solemn affairs; there was never a witticism or light moment; the burden of the matter hung upon him like a cloud which sobered us into rapt attention. They were a strange contrast to other lectures; the quiet, order, and attention placed them in a class by themselves.

Medical students in those days were fuller of animal spirits which at times boisterously overflowed; they loved to indulge in meaningless applause, and some of the professors had little control over the men. Occasionally a lecturer would lose his temper and leave the class; but the fiasco was ere long repeated and had a way of culminating at periodic intervals.

There was no meaning in it and it depended in some mysterious way upon the personality of the lecturer. Men of character commanded audience, but the weaklings succumbed, especially those who did not take the bull by the horns at the opening of the session. Naturally they were more in evidence in the junior courses, but even in the senior they never quite disappeared.

Some curious and amusing incidents occurred and I could say much upon the subject, but I only mention it to show the contrast to the way in which Lister was treated. A pin-drop could be heard in his presence; he riveted attention and cast a spell of seriousness and earnestness over all. Once and once only was it broken.

61

The Professor had entered the theatre in his usual thoughtful and solemn manner, followed by the clerk who was carrying the spray. Chatter immediately ceased and dead silence ensued, when suddenly from the top of the theatre, in sonorous and clerical tones, a voice was heard: 'Let us s-pray!' Every one appreciated the humour but we were too staggered even to smile. Slowly Lister raised his eyes to the speaker with sad and pitying glance without uttering a word! The effect was magical, the most oppressive silence followed and work was resumed. A year later the man died of general paralysis; we knew nothing then of spirochetes [the bacteria responsible for syphilis] and it was playfully suggested Jove had smitten him for the sacrilege!

William Ernest Henley *Letter to Harry Nichols, September 1873*

Saturday 23rd August is my twenty-fourth birthday; parritch and buttermilk, dry bread and corfey – boiled beef and cabbage (ugh!) tea and dry bread – buttermilk.* Thursday 28th. I go to seek a great Perhaps. I get into a basket borne by four students. 'Gentlemen, have a care! You carry Caesar and his fortunes!'

---

* Henley was obviously not enamoured of the Infirmary diet. Margaret Mathewson raised no such complaints: maybe food in Shetland was less varied and less substantial than in London. R. J. S. McDowall in his classic exposition of the delights of whisky, also enthuses about the Infirmary's porridge:

> Most readers of this book will probably not know that the flavour of porridge made from oatmeal and water flavoured with salt varies greatly according to the speed with which it is boiled. Steaming all night before it is eaten as done in Edinburgh Royal Infirmary probably makes the best porridge.[26]

BEFORE in *Poems* (1898)

Behold me waiting – waiting for the knife.
A little while, and at a leap I storm
The thick, sweet mystery of chloroform,
The drunken dark, the little death-in-life.
The gods are good to me: I have no wife,
No innocent child, to think of as I near
The fateful minute; nothing all-too dear
Unmans me for my bout of passive strife.
Yet am I tremulous and a trifle sick,
And, face to face with chance, I shrink a little:
My hopes are strong, my will is something weak.
Here comes the basket? Thank you. I am ready.
But, gentlemen my porters, life is brittle:
You carry Caesar and his fortunes – steady!

Margaret Mathewson   *Sketch*

Just then I was called upstairs and sat three hours in the
dark hole. Then I was not wanted after all. In going up the
Lobby, I met Dr. Cheyne. He came laughing and said
'Oh, I'm glad to see you stood your operation so well
today.'

I said 'Yes thank you sir, I stood it fine, I think.'

'Were you cold in the dark hole all yon hours?'

'Yes sir, I was cold and hungry too, but I see I am like
the lawyer and the barber, I have got to wait.'

He laughed and enjoyed the lark very well (next day I
got dinner).

I went into No. 3 when all shout 'Oh, look, here's
Maggie back again without anything done yet. Well, we
really thought you were getting your goose cooked today.'

'No, Prof. has let me off this time yet as they know I
won't run far away.'

I got a lot of teasing about going upstairs so often, but it
was all in lark, and if it was my turn then, it would be some
of theirs next. However I was called upstairs every day for
a fortnight and thus fear had given place to confidence.

Everyday of this fortnight my dinner was kept off and I was getting thin.

Then brother Arthur came from Campbeltown on his way home. He had been there 6 months with brother Walter, who is a Lightkeeper there. Arthur expected I would get home with him after a week or a fortnight longer in the Infirmary. Thus he waited for me and came every evening at visiting hours, and it passed the time much better, but I never told him how serious I really expected the operation to be as I thought he would be writing Father, and they all would get anxious. But a fortnight previously Dr. Cheyne had written Rev. Barclay stating the nature of my operation. This Mr. Barclay went and told Father. Thus my friends at home knew about it before I was aware.

On March 23rd Dr. Cheyne came into No. 3 after breakfast and asked me 'Have you had breakfast?'

'Yes, sir.'

'Not a big one, I hope?'

'I had the usual quantity sir, and the way I get no dinner I think I would require a big one.'

He went away laughing but I dreaded there was a different kind of dinner preparing for me today and about 10.30 a.m. Nurse Kilpatrick came and told me to undress as usual and be quick as I would soon be called, but it was 1 p.m. ere Dr. Cheyne came and called me. We passed up through the crowded stair as most of the students were returning to college. The big theatre door was open and we went in. Prof. bowed and smiled. I returned the bow. He then told me to step up on the chair (set at the side of the table on which was a blanket and 2 pillows) then lie down on the table. I did so and saw that my turn had come at last and now was the time to be cool and as collected as possible – as my anxiety will not alter Prof's intentions.

There were a lot sitting in the gallery and four gentlemen sitting around the table. Dr. Cheyne came and laid a towel saturated with chloroform over my face and said 'Now breathe away.' I then felt Professor's hand laid gently on my arm as if to let me know he was near me, which I could and did confide in and this did encourage me to hope for the best. I then breathed a few sentences of silent earnest prayer. Then the precious text came to mind: 'Fear thou not for I am with thee; Be not dismayed, for I am thy God. I will strengthen thee; Yea I will help

64

thee; yea I will uphold thee with the right hand of my righteousness.' Isaiah 41.10.

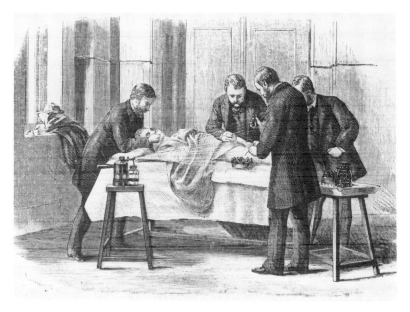

A model antiseptic operation using the spray. Note the attire of the doctors. (BBC Hulton Picture Library)

I felt myself growing weaker and weaker and every nerve and joint relaxing and breaking up as it were, a very solemn moment thus staring death in the face and I believed I never should awaken to look on the things of time any more but was indeed entering eternity. I then thought this must be the valley of the shadow of death I am now passing through. 'Yea, though I walk through the valley of the shadow of death, I will fear no evil; for thou art with me, thy rod and thy staff, they comfort me.'

I then bade goodbye to each friend, though no relative was near, but I felt Jesus was near and a very present help in time of trouble.

William Ernest Henley

OPERATION in *Poems* (1898)

You are carried in a basket,
Like a carcase from the shambles,
To the theatre, a cockpit
Where they stretch you on a table.

Then they bid you close your eyelids,
And they mask you with a napkin,
And the anaesthetic reaches
Hot and subtle through your being.

And you gasp and reel and shudder
In a rushing, swaying rapture,
While the voices at your elbow
Fade – receding – fainter – farther.

Lights about you shower and tumble,
And your blood seems crystallising –
Edged and vibrant, yet within you
Racked and hurried back and forward.

Then the lights grow fast and furious,
And you hear a noise of waters,
And you wrestle, blind and dizzy,
In an agony of effort.

Till a sudden lull accepts you,
And you sound an utter darkness . . .
And awaken . . . with a struggle . . .
On a hushed attentive audience.

Henley's return to consciousness was much more civilized than some. In an undated letter, Margaret describes a rather ruder awakening. The doctor referred to is Patrick Heron Watson, a contemporary of Lister, and an eminent surgeon:

> . . . Dr. Watson had the first case of 3 of the same and his patient died in the chloroform. Next one Professor Lister

got and cured and when the person awoke (in the Theatre) all the students got up and applauded him. I think Dr. Watson was there too . . .

William Ernest Henley   *Letter to Harry Nichols, September 1873*

Out of chloroform, I find my foot is still *all there*. Saturday, 30th August, the Professor says, 'You can write and tell your friends that I have done what I could and that I am perfectly satisfied.' Since then, going on as well as possible. For the present, therefore, my foot is SAVED!!!

Margaret Mathewson   *Sketch*

I was conscious of no more until I awoke in bed in a strange ward, viz. No. 2. My first thought was 'My arm is it off or not?' I at once sat up to feel for it. I could not find it at all, but I was all bandaged up from the waist to the neck. It must be away.

I then found it bandaged to my waist and breathed a sigh of thankfulness to God for this renewed instance of His goodness to me. Some of the patients had shouted for the nurse to come to me. She came in agitation on seeing me sitting up. 'Maggie, what are you doing? You must lie down at once, like a good girl.'

'I was looking for my arm, Nurse, to see if it was here or not.'

'Oh, yes, it is here still Maggie. Now, lie down and go asleep.'

I did so and slept about half an hour.

John Rudd Leeson   *Lister as I Knew Him*

The operating theatre was grimed with the filth of decades; I suppose it was occasionally cleaned, but such process was never in evidence. There was but one window, the large one to the north, which lighted it, but it was never opened. The frayed old wooden floor was browny-red telling its tale of the scenes it had witnessed. Many of the students came straight from the dissecting room. The operating table, looked as though it was never washed and around its base sawdust was sprinkled. A semi-circle of hair-stuffed chairs that had seen years of service were placed around the front of the arena and were generally occupied by foreign professors who had come to see and study the new treatment.

The entrance of Lister into the theatre is a memory that cannot be forgotten: his impressive presence and arresting personality, his anxious, thoughtful, and beneficent face lit up by his sweetly observant and commanding eyes, which worked with his mobile lips in revealing thought as his mind evolved action.

Four satellites accompanied him: the house surgeon, apprehensive and fidgety lest any dresser or clerk should fail in duty; the instrument clerk, carrying the tray on which were arranged the instruments, always scrupulously covered with a towel – or woe betide him; the clerk with the spray, fearful lest a full head of steam should not be immediately available, twiddling about with the spirit-lamp to make sure he was getting the best out of it; and the chloroform clerk, with his bottles and towel, and tongue-forceps dangling from his coat-lappet.

After a kindly smile of greeting to his audience the Professor seated himself on the old worn horsehair-covered chair which had served as the chair of clinical surgery for generations and must have been a museum of microbes, cast a towel over his left knee, heaved the accustomed little sigh and began his lecture.

In front of him stood the operating table, a plain kitchen table devoid of all accessories, upon an old wooden floor frayed with wear and stained with years of blood, upon which were sprinkled a few handfuls of sawdust; at the side of the window was a large leaden sink, but there were no basins or other provision for the washing of hands.

No one dreamt of washing his hands before commencing work. I have seen dressers assisting who wore 'mourning' beneath their nails. No one ever took off his coat; occasionally the professor would turn up his cuffs, but the assistants never; probably they would have considered it a breach of etiquette as assuming an unwarranted importance.

Lister had tried water, soap and cleanliness in Glasgow, but without practical results, and this, in part, drove him on to his antiseptic regimen. He became so confident about carbolic that he subsequently neglected mere hygiene. One of Lister's house surgeons wrote that Lister himself wore 'an old blue frock-coat for operations, which he had previously worn in the dissecting room. It was stiff and glazed with blood.'[27] The 'or woe betide him' in Leeson's account above refers to another story:

One day the instrument clerk so far forgot himself that he brought the instrument tray into the theatre – *uncovered!*
Lister at once detected it and instantly threw a towel over the tray, and turning to the clerk said in slow and sorrowful tones: 'How can you have such cruel disregard for this poor woman's feelings? Is it not enough for her to be passing through this ordeal without adding unnecessarily to her sufferings by displaying this array of naked steel? Really, Mr. __, I am surprised at you.'

Further on, Leeson tells a similar story, at his own expense:

. . . when all was ready Lister turned to me, his face wearing the usual look of careworn earnestness, and said, 'A knife please, Mr. Leeson,' and I handed him a scalpel. He carefully, as was his wont, tested its edge upon the palm of his hand, found it defective, and solemnly and slowly walked across the ward and put it upon the fire.

Retracing his steps to his former position, in exactly the same tones he repeated his request: 'A knife please, Mr. Leeson.'

I handed him another scalpel; again he tried its edge, and again walked to the fire and placed it upon the coals.

The scene can be better imagined than described. The patients were amazed at the extraordinary sight of the Professor burning his instruments; the students were galvanised to attention, glancing now at Lister, then at me, and those on the outskirts of the crowd suddenly aroused to extraordinary curiosity to discover what it was all about. The foreigners seemed utterly mystified; there was much that was novel in antiseptic ritual, but the burning of knives overpassed all.

Lister solemnly walked back to his old position, and for the third time in exactly the same tones, said, 'A knife please, Mr. Leeson.' With fear and trembling, and hardly knowing what I was doing, I handed him a third scalpel. He tested it like the others, and to my joy and relief it passed muster. He then slowly raised his eyes, and looking me full in the face quietly and deliberately said, 'Thank you, that will do'; and then after a pause drew an unusually deep breath, as though to nerve himself for the effort, and with an expression I shall never forget, said, 'Mr. Leeson, how dare you hand me a knife to use upon this poor man that you would not like to have used upon yourself?'

Leeson finds Lister's deep concern for his patients praise-worthy, but Fisher notes judiciously that, while such gestures make splendid operating-room *theatre*, a private word with the culprit would have been rather less terrifying for the patient – as well as less humiliating for the poor clerk or dresser.[28]

Lister's attitude to his patients was one of high Victorian paternalism: one suspects he wished to improve surgery more than help people live better lives. He once said of his long-stay patients 'Who knows, it may be that whilst here they may have a chance of learning something of the meaning of the word Gratitude.'[29]

Arthur Conan Doyle was a medical student in Edinburgh from 1876 to 1881 and wrote a splendid short story about a young student's initiation in the rites of surgery:[30]

Arthur Conan Doyle   *His First Operation*

It was the first day of a winter session, and the third year's man was walking with the first year's man. Twelve o'clock just booming out from the Tron Church.

'Let me see,' said the third year's man, 'you have never seen an operation?'

'Never.'

'Then this way, please. This is Rutherford's historic bar. A glass of sherry, please, for this gentleman. You are rather sensitive, are you not?'

'My nerves are not very strong, I am afraid.'

'Hum! Another glass of sherry for this gentleman. We are going to an operation now, you know.'

The novice squared his shoulders and made a gallant attempt to look unconcerned.

'Nothing very bad – eh?'

'Well, yes – pretty bad.'

'An – an amputation?'

'No, it's a bigger affair than that.'

'I think – I think they must be expecting me at home.'

'There's no sense funking. If you don't go today you must tomorrow. Better get it over at once. Feel pretty fit?'

'Oh, yes, all right.'

The smile was not a success.

'One more glass of sherry, then. Now come on or we shall be late. I want you to be well in front.'

'Surely that is not necessary.'

'Oh, it is far better. What a drove of students! There are plenty of new men among them. You can tell them easily enough, can't you? If they were going down to be operated upon themselves they could not look whiter.'

'I don't think I should look as white.'

'Well, I was just the same myself. But the feeling soon wears off. You see a fellow with a face like plaster, and before the week is out he is eating his lunch in the dissecting rooms. I'll tell you all about the case when we get to the theatre.'

The students were pouring down the sloping street which led to the infirmary – each with his little sheaf of notebooks in his hand. There were pale, frightened lads, fresh from the High Schools, and callous old chronics, whose generation had passed on and left them. They

71

swept in an unbroken, tumultuous stream from the University gate to the hospital. The figures and gait of the men were young, but there was little youth in most of their faces. Some looked as if they ate too little – a few as if they drank too much. Tall and short, tweed coated and black, round-shouldered, bespectacled and slim, they crowded with clatter of feet and rattle of sticks through the hospital gate. Now and again they thickened into two lines as the carriage of a surgeon of the staff rolled over the cobble-stones between.

'There's going to be a crowd at Archer's,' whispered the senior man with suppressed excitement. 'It is grand to see him at work. I've seen him jab all round the aorta until it made me jumpy to watch him. This way, and mind the whitewash.'

They passed under an archway and down a long, stone-flagged corridor with drab coloured doors on either side, each marked with a number. Some of them were ajar, and the novice glanced into them with tingling nerves. He was reassured to catch a glimpse of cheery fires, lines of white-counterpaned beds and a profusion of coloured texts upon the wall. The corridor opened upon a small hall with a fringe of poorly-clad people seated all round upon benches. A young man with a pair of scissors stuck, like a flower, in his button-hole, and a notebook in his hand, was passing from one to the other, whispering and writing.

'Anything good?' asked the third year's man.

'You should have been here yesterday,' said the out-patient clerk, glancing up. 'We had a regular field day. A popliteal aneurysm, a Colles' fracture, a spina bifida, a tropical abscess, and an elephantiasis. How's that for a single haul?'

'I'm sorry I missed it. But they'll come again, I suppose. What's up with the old gentleman?'

A broken workman was sitting in the shadow, rocking himself slowly to and fro and groaning. A woman beside him was trying to console him, patting his shoulder with a hand which was spotted over with curious little white blisters.

'It's a fine carbuncle,' said the clerk, with the air of a connoisseur who describes his orchids to one who can appreciate them. 'It's on his back, and the passage is draughty, so we must not look at it, must we, daddy? Pemphigus,' he added carelessly, pointing to the woman's

72

disfigured hands. 'Would you care to stop and take out a metacarpal?'

'No thank you, we are due at Archer's. Come on;' and they rejoined the throng which was hurrying to the theatre of the famous surgeon.

The tiers of horseshoe benches, rising from the floor to the ceiling, were already packed, and the novice as he entered saw vague, curving lines of faces in front of him, and heard the deep buzz of a hundred voices and sounds of laughter from somewhere up above him. His companion spied an opening on the second bench, and they both squeezed into it.

'This is grand,' the senior man whispered; 'you'll have a rare view of it all.'

Only a single row of heads intervened between them and the operating table. It was of unpainted deal, plain, strong and scrupulously clean. A sheet of brown water-proofing covered half of it, and beneath stood a large tin tray full of sawdust. On the further side, in front of the window, there was a board which was strewed with glittering instruments, forceps, tenacula, saws, canulas and trocars. A line of knives, with long, thin, delicate blades, lay at one side. Two young men lounged in front of this; one threading needles, the other doing something to a brass coffee-pot-like thing which hissed out puffs of steam.

'That's Peterson,' whispered the senior. 'The big, bald man in the front row. He's the skin-grafting man, you know. And that's Anthony Browne, who took a larynx out successfully last winter. And there's Murphy the path-ologist, and Stoddart the eye man. You'll come to know them all soon.'

'Who are the two men at the table?'

'Nobody – dressers. One has charge of the instruments and the other of the puffing Billy. It's Lister's antiseptic spray, you know, and Archer's one of the carbolic acid men. Hayes is the leader of the cleanliness-and-cold-water school, and they all hate each other like poison.'

A flutter of interest passed through the closely-packed benches as a woman in petticoat and bodice was led in by two nurses. A red wollen shawl was draped over her head and round her neck. The face which looked out from it was that of a woman in the prime of her years, but drawn with suffering and of a peculiar bees-wax tint. Her head drooped as she walked, and one of the nurses, with her arm round her waist, was whispering consolation in her ear. She gave a quick side glance at the instrument table as she passed, but the nurses turned her away from it.

'What ails her?' asked the novice.

'Cancer of the parotid. It's the devil of a case, extends right away back behind the carotids. There's hardly a man but Archer would dare to follow it. Ah, here he is himself.'

As he spoke, a small brisk, iron-grey man came striding into the room, rubbing his hands together as he walked. He had a clean-shaven face of the naval officer type, with large, bright eyes, and a firm, straight mouth. Behind him came his big house surgeon with his gleaming pince-nez and a trail of dressers, who grouped themselves into the corners of the room.

'Gentlemen,' cried the surgeon in a voice as hard and brisk as his manner. 'We have here an interesting case of tumour of the parotid, originally cartilaginous but now assuming malignant characteristics, and therefore requiring excision. On to the table, nurse! Thank you! Chloroform, clerk! Thank you! You can take the shawl off, nurse.'

The woman lay back upon the waterproofed pillow and her murderous tumour lay revealed. In itself it was a pretty thing, ivory white with a mesh of blue veins, and curving gently from jaw to chest. But the lean, yellow face, and the stringy throat were in horrible contrast with the plumpness and sleekness of this monstrous growth. The surgeon placed a hand on each side of it and pressed it slowly backwards and forwards.

'Adherent at one place, gentlemen,' he cried. 'The growth involves the carotids and jugulars, and passes behind the ramus of the jaw, whither we must be prepared to follow it. It is impossible to say how deep our dissection may carry us. Carbolic tray, thank you! Dressings of carbolic gauze, if you please! Push the chloroform, Mr. Johnson. Have the small saw ready in case it is necessary to remove the jaw.'

The patient was moaning gently under the towel which had been placed over her face. She tried to raise her arms and to draw up her knees but two dressers restrained her. The heavy air was full of the penetrating smells of carbolic acid and of chloroform. A muffled cry came from under the towel and then a snatch of a song, sung in a high, quavering, monotonous voice.

> He says, says he,
> If you fly with me
>> You'll be mistress of the ice-cream van;
>> You'll be mistress of the –

It mumbled off into a drone and stopped. The surgeon came across, still rubbing his hands, and spoke to an elderly man in front of the novice.

'Narrow squeak for the Government,' he said.

'Oh, ten is enough.'

'They won't have ten long. They'd do better to resign before they are driven to it.'

'Oh, I should fight it out.'

'What's the use. They can't get past the committee, even if they get a vote in the House. I was talking to –'

'Patient's ready, sir,' said the dresser.

'Talking to M'Donald – but I'll tell you about it presently.'

He walked back to the patient, who was breathing in long, heavy gasps. 'I propose', said he, passing his hand over the tumour in an almost caressing fashion, 'to make a free incision over the posterior border and to take another forward at right angles to the lower end of it. Might I trouble you for a medium knife, Mr. Johnson.'

The novice, with eyes which were dilating with horror, saw the surgeon pick up the long, gleaming knife, dip it into a tin basin and balance it in his fingers as an artist might his brush. Then he saw him pinch up the skin above the tumour with his left hand. At the sight, his nerves, which had already been tried once or twice that day, gave way utterly. His head swam round and he felt that in another instant he might faint. He dared not look at the patient. He dug his thumbs into his ears less some scream should come to haunt him, and he fixed his eyes rigidly upon the wooden ledge in front of him. One glance, one cry, would, he knew, break down the shred of self-possession which he still retained. He tried to think of cricket, of green fields and rippling water, of his sisters at home – of anything rather than of what was going on so near him.

And yet, somehow, even with his ears stopped up, sounds seemed to penetrate to him and to carry their own tale. He heard, or thought he heard, the long hissing of the carbolic engine. Then he was conscious of some movement among the dressers. Were there groans too breaking in upon him, and some other sound, some fluid sound which was more dreadfully suggestive still? His mind would keep building up every step of the operation, and fancy made it more ghastly than fact could have been. His nerves tingled and quivered. Minute by minute the giddiness grew more marked, the numb, sickly feeling at his heart more distressing. And then suddenly, with a groan, his head pitching forward and his brow cracking sharply upon the narrow, wooden shelf in front of him, he lay in a dead faint.

When he came to himself he was lying in the empty theatre with his collar and shirt undone. The third year's man was dabbing a wet sponge over his face, and a couple of grinning dressers were looking on.

'All right,' cried the novice, sitting up and rubbing his eyes; 'I'm sorry to have made an ass of myself.'

'Well, so I should think,' said his companion. 'What on earth did you faint about?'

'I couldn't help it. It was that operation.'

'What operation?'

'Why, that cancer.'

There was a pause, and then the three students burst out laughing.

'Why, you juggins,' cried the senior man, 'there never was an operation at all. They found the patient didn't stand the chloroform well, and so the whole thing was off. Archer has been giving us one of his racy lectures, and you fainted just in the middle of his favourite story.'

This story draws very closely on Conan Doyle's experiences as a medical student in Edinburgh. Hayes – the enemy of antiseptic surgery – was in reality James Spence, another Edinburgh Professor, while Archer, the adherent of antiseptics, was Joseph Bell, one of Lister's colleagues.

Bell has traditionally been held as the model Arthur Conan Doyle used for Sherlock Holmes. In his autobiography, *Memories and Adventures*, Conan Doyle quotes an example of Bell's deductive skills:

Arthur Conan Doyle   *Memories and Adventures*

In one of his best cases he said to a civilian patient:
'Well, my man, you've served in the army.'
'Aye, sir.'
'Not long discharged?'
'No, sir.'
'A Highland regiment?'
'Aye, sir.'
'A non-com. officer?'
'Aye, sir.'
'Stationed at Barbados?'
'Aye, sir.'
'You see, gentlemen,' he would explain, 'the man was a respectful man but did not remove his hat. They do not in the army, but he would have learned civilian ways had he been long discharged. He has an air of authority and he is obviously Scottish. As to Barbados, his complaint is elephantiasis, which is West Indian not British.' To his audience of Watsons it all seemed very miraculous until it was explained, and then it became simple enough.[31]

In *The Quest for Sherlock Holmes* (Edinburgh, 1983), Owen Dudley Edwards has shown that in fact the provenance of Sherlock Holmes is not so simple, and that Conan Doyle used aspects of many of his friends and acquaintances in the Edinburgh medical community to build his detective's character.

Margaret Mathewson   *Sketch*

When I awoke nurse was bringing in the tea at 4.30 p.m. as usual. I dozed over again then heard them with the dishes then looked up and saw nurse gathering them on a tray and Arthur came in. I at once sat up to speak to him but felt I had to vomit. I looked for the solution pan. It was on the quilt at my elbow. I held out my hand to Arthur but could not speak for vomiting. He had only sitten about

5 minutes when Miss Logan came to him and said, 'Please we can't allow any visitors in this ward tonight, as Margaret is so weak, also a wee baby there at the fire.'

He at once said Good night, and a ticket was put on the door 'No Visitors allowed'. This baby was brought in with a 'heir shire lip', also 'bronchitis' and got his operation the same day that I did. His lip was sewed up, the throat cut, and the bronchial tubes scraped and cleaned. He was only 6 weeks old and was an admirable case. At the two months end he was dismissed 'cured'.*

Now to return to my own feelings and treatment. I felt very sick and kept on vomiting. The nurse brought a jug of ice and gave me always a teaspoonful as soon as I stopped vomiting. 'This ice will give me toothache if I eat much of it, nurse.'

'Oh, no it won't. You must eat a lot, Maggie, as it will do your wounds good and help you on quicker.'

I got more feverish and sick, and felt the vomiting more – straining on the stomack, and always grew weaker. Dr. Cheyne came and took my pulse, marked it down on the card. Miss Logan came at every half hour and took my pulse. I asked her 'If you please Miss Logan did you get my watch and purse from Mary Ann in No. 3?'

'Yes.'

'Well, please when you roll the watch, it rolls the opposite way of yours.'

'Very well and I'll keep it for you a few days.'

'Thank you Miss Logan.'

I vomited all the evening now and again. I went asleep but soon awoke and felt more feverish, also a bad headache, a strange pain about the joint and smarting all around as if it were cut. As the night wore on the pain increased, and at times I was on the eve of shouting, the pain was so severe. I then thought 'I shall not shout as long as I can avoid it.' I thus hid my mouth in the sheet. I felt giddy and asked Nurse for another pillow and got it as I fancied I would not feel so sick. But it was the same.

---

* With antiseptics, it was now reasonable for Lister to perform plastic surgery on a hare-lip; no longer was it laughable to perform such strictly unnecessary operations (see p. 1).

I felt so warm, I put down the quilt. Nurse said 'No you must not put off the quilt, but keep chewing ice – that will keep you cool. Would you have a drink?'

'Yes nurse please.'

Nurse went and she seemed a long time away. She must be putting on a fire some place and yet she is special nurse for the baby and I. She can't be there likely she will be upstairs speaking to the Dr. Just then she returned with a medicine glass of morphia, laudanum etc. She told me to take this quite up, and it would better me. I was not inclined to take it at all, as I had seen the effects of similar drafts on others.

She persuaded me, and told me 'It would ease the pain which you are trying to choke every now and then.' I took it.

Passing 2 a.m. I felt very sleepy but could not go asleep for the starting pain around the joint, as if the arm was flying off from my body altogether. About 3 a.m. I went asleep, and slept until 5.30 a.m. when nurse was making the beds. She came and said 'Do you feel any better. You have had a nice sleep?'

'Yes thank you I feel a little better. I have had a good sleep.'

I soon had to vomit and at intervals vomited for hours. Nurse McDougal kept feeding me with ice now and again.

'When are you going to stop vomiting?'

'I don't know. I doubt it will be sometime ere I get over this horrid chloroform taste and its effects.'

In a little the Dr. came and took my pulse and put down 120 point 4 on the card. He asked 'What like is your pain?'

'I feel it sore, but not painful at present sir.'

'That's singular.'

'Well sir, that's how I feel it at present.'

At 11 a.m. Professor came in and asked 'How are you this morning?'

'Thank you, sir, but I feel very weak.'

'Yes, you must be weak, but I will soon be coming to dress you and then it will feel better.'

About 12.45 Professor came and a train of students with him. He asked 'Do you now find any pain?'

'Yes sir.'

'What like is it? Is it a severe pain, an acute pain, an aching pain or starting pain?'

'It is neither sir, it is a squeezing pain as if it was squeezed with a cord sir.'

'Yes, so it is. Are you able to sit up and I will now dress it.'

I tried to do so but fell back on the pillow. Two students then helped me up. Professor asked 'How was it you loosened the bandages?' Dr. Cheyne said 'That was in the chloroform, sir and thus she does not know and therefore we must excuse her.'

'Yes. Well, will you promise me never to undo the bandages again and if you feel any way uncomfortable just tell Miss Logan.'

'Yes, sir I will.'

Prof. then dressed it with the spray, then put on chloride of zinc and moved the arm to and fro. The pain was indescribable. I never felt such excruciating pain before. I also felt the arm quite loose from my body. The pain caused me almost to faint.

Prof. said to the students: 'Gentlemen, I have a great fear of putrefaction setting in and you all know its outcome. Thus I will look anxiously for the second day or third day between hope and fear. I hope the chloride of zinc will preserve it but it is only an experiment. However we will see if spared.'

By now Lister was committed to carbolic acid, but he continued to try out many compounds recommended to him by doctors, chemists or others, hoping to find the ideal antiseptic, a powerful germicide that would not be mortifying to the flesh. Amongst the chemicals he tried were: salicylic acid (the important ingredient in aspirin!), thymol, eucalyptus (both of which were volatile, but this advantage was offset by practical difficulties), corrosive sublimate, sal alembroth, double cyanide of mercury and zinc (he tested a whole group of mercury's compounds) and boracic acid (already in use as a meat-preservative and though the weakest germicide on the list, the only one still in use). Spectators at Lister's operations were often curious about the little bits of gauze that were seen festooning his arm if and when he rolled his sleeves up. These were, in fact, various antiseptic compounds soaked at various strengths into bandages and applied to his own flesh to see how irritating they were.

Zinc chloride, however, was not among these. Its use in wound dressings was well established (see p. 10), and the conversation Margaret Mathewson reports here is, presumably, a piece of self-dramatization.

Margaret Mathewson   *Sketch*

I thought over the last of Professor's speech seriously. Evidently he has very poor hopes of my recovery indeed. I thus better now look over my hopes of eternity, where probably I will soon be in reality and see if my hope will stand the test of 'The Judgement Day'.

While I was thus thinking Miss Logan came and had stood a little at the bedside ere I observed her. She said 'Margaret what are you thinking on?'

'On what the Professor said.'

'Well I daresay, but you must eat as much ice as ever you can as your life depends on how much ice you eat. Never mind how often the jug is done, just you eat as much as you can and you may get better.'

She then took my pulse and came back every half hour for the same, then every quarter of an hour and I saw both the Dr. and nurse seemed anxious and thoughtful and I believed were dreading 12 o'clock's approach as they looked often to their watches. I thought 'It's I that has the most cause to be anxious and thoughtful, who am evidently on the verge of another world.'

As 12 p.m. approached I grew worse and weaker. Then Satan came with his word of comfort. 'You have the dark valley of death to pass through ere you get to heaven and who will help you then?'

'God will as he has said: "Lo, I am with you always even unto the end of the world." Yea though I walk through the valley of the shadow of death, I will fear no evil for thou art with me, thy rod and thy staff they comfort me.'

'But will he stand to that?'

81

'Yes he will for he has said: "Fear thou not for I am with thee, be not dismayed for I am thy God I will strengthen thee, yea I will help thee, yea I will uphold thee with the right hand of my righteousness."' And Satan then left me.

The vomiting still kept up and I grew very weak but felt humbly thankful I had not now in a dying hour to grapple with Satan under the weight of my sins. I then fancied all my friends at home around me. I pressed on each one to make sure work for eternity, of having peace with God through Jesus alone and then we should all meet again on the other side of the river as I felt sure Jesus was coming to take me to be for ever with himself. I then bade everyone 'Goodbye' which was a painful parting indeed.

Then the dark valley burst on my imagination and as it were a river before me, which I was about to drop into, yet a natural feeling of shrinking back on seeing the waves running so high. 'It is impossible I can get over those waves.'

'Fear not for I am with thee' I thought I heard a voice say and I looked to see my guide, when I saw a person clothed in white, and he smiled and held out his hand. I recognised him at once to be Jesus himself. I grasped his hand and on looking to the river again instantly it changed into dry ground as it were an earthen pavement. But it seemed still dark and we went on it and it continued dark a short time. But I felt no fear as Jesus was with me and holding my hand, and then it instantly became all light and continued and continued increasing until I thought 'What a beautiful sunshine' and it seemed to dazzle my sight when I thought Jesus said to me 'Look, do you see this gate?'

'Yes.'

And I kept my eye on it and I believed this was the gate of heaven and we were quite near it, and expected it to open as we stood at it, when Jesus looked to me and smiled saying 'You cannot go further at present but must return for a little longer and tell more sinners the way of salvation.'

I felt indeed sad to hear this, as altho' my lifetime had not been long (only 28 years) yet I had found it made up of many things which had been very trying, so many years of pain and suffering.

Then Jesus (who knows even the thoughts of the heart) said 'Lo, I am with you always even to the end of the world.'

I said 'Not my will but thine be done, O Lord', and I felt no dread to face whatever might be before me through the 'little longer' I would have in time. I thus felt encouraged to return and begin life afresh, with a redoubled energy to work with a greater object in view than heretofore. We returned to the other side of the river and I looked before me when I again beheld my friends around me, welcoming me back to their bosoms with such extasy. I opened my eyes and lo! I was in the Infirmary ward!!

The perspiration was running down my forehead, and I was all wet with it and so weak and dry. I saw the nurse at another bed and tried to ask her for a drink but I could not speak out over, so I put my fingers into the ice jug on the table and lifted some drops to my mouth. Then the nurse looked round and I held up my hand to her. She came running 'Oh, I am glad to see you awake so fresh.'

'Awake nurse, why I have not been asleep.'

'Oh, yes, you have.'

'Please nurse, give me just a good drink, not those bits of ice any longer, as I do feel so thirsty.'

'No, no, I can't do that as you would take too much, but those bits of ice is both your food and drink for a time yet, Maggie. I have nursed many patients but I never before met with one who could eat ice like you. You surely must have been born at the north pole among the ice Maggie.'

'No, nurse, not quite at the pole, but the next land to it.'

Then the Dr. came in.

'Well nurse is she awake yet?'

'Oh yes sir and she's much better.'

'Yes, I hope she will [improve] now. Do you feel any better?'

'Yes sir, but very weak.'

'Yes you must feel weak.' He took my pulse.

'Oh you are a lot better, your pulse is down 20 points since I was in ¾ of an hour ago.'

Soon after I went asleep and slept a good while, and on awakening I began again to vomit (which kept up some weeks at intervals). The nurse came, and sat down, and asked me 'What was it you were dreaming that time when you awoke so weak? You talked like a parson talking to an unconverted person. Then you said Goodbye for ever in this life to a lot of friends, and the tears were coursing down your cheeks. But a little after you seemed so calm and happy and again talking to a familiar friend which seemed to be going with you some way or to some place. I really thought you were dying and I called the Doctor. He watched you closely for ¾ of an hour on his watch and said "It is the turning point either for life or death." Your pulse was the highest he has seen unless a fever case. It was 150 point 4 put down there on the card. He kept watching you until he found the pulse go down 20 points then said "She's now over the worst and I am very glad as it is such an interesting case."'

I was aroused by Professor Lister coming in so early as 9 a.m. instead of 11 a.m. He as usual made a courtesy and seemed so glad, holding out his hand to me and said, 'Well, I am thankful to see you looking so well this morning. How are you?'

'Thank you sir, I feel much better, but very weak.'

'Yes, you must be weak for sometime yet but I will be coming to dress you soon and then you will feel the arm easier.'

'Thank you sir.' He then folded his hands, closed his eyes in silent prayer, stood a few minutes thus, then again bowed and went out.

About 11.45 Prof. came to dress me and a great many students. When Prof. had taken off the bandages, he said, 'Gentlemen to my glad surprise you see there's neither colour nor smell here and it is preserved entirely by the chloride of zinc.'

'How much of it did you use sir?' asked a Dr. '2/3rds. I hope it will yet come to be a useful arm.'

Prof. then moved it (which caused excruciating pain and ever after I dreaded the moving). Prof. then bandaged it up, then said, 'Gentlemen, I had great fears of the patient standing the operation, as her constitution was so reduced by the daily use of internal medicines for about 3 years, and severe suffering from several diseases being in the system all at once, which adds to its singularity. She took a very small quantity of chloroform at first only about ½ an ounce, but that was not near enough to keep her quiet, the time I required for the operation. Thus I had to repeat the dose often until I feared to give more for getting her back. And after all it required an hour and ten minutes to restore her, and it's effects must have been heavy and will be felt for some time yet to come, but I trust it will now be a successful case.'

Lister's attack on the 'daily use of internal medicines' is an attack on the patent medicines purveyed unscrupulously and very profitably in the nineteenth century. For Margaret, stuck in the Shetlands, it must have been difficult to resist the adverts for some of these elixirs of life. On 20 December 1876, we find her writing to her brother:

> The stuff I got from H.H. did no good worth speaking of – during the time I used it in fact I rather felt worse. The two pills which was sent with the medicine was to be taken both at once, my word, I wont meddle with his pills in a hurry again and the place (the shoulder joint and a little below) I rubbed the stuff on has swelled up like a little pudden . . .

She also consulted with the apothecary in Aberdeen who stocked these patent cures, asking him for medical advice on her condition:

> . . . I also had Mr. Horrells answer and 32 powders on Monday night, but he says he can scarcely say what's to do with my arm, but says something to rub in at night might do it some good, but if it does not improve from the powders (which is for chest, liver etc.) he wishes me to write him again.

And well he might.

While some of these nostrums contained unpredictable quantities of dangerous drugs, others contained nothing: Rollos Remedy for Piles on analysis proved to consist of 99 per cent fat and a 'small quantity of very dark stuff'![32] Dangerous or no, they all cost exhorbitant sums of money which would have been much better spent on proper food or warmth. The use of chloroform was dangerous, and these dangers were exacerbated by Margaret's enfeebled constitution.

In antiseptic surgery, the surgeon's job did not begin and end with the operation. He also had to keep the wound germ-free before and after the operation. The trouble Lister took in bandaging his patients marked him out from other surgeons.

John Rudd Leeson *Lister as I Knew Him*

He always applied the operation dressings himself; they were invariably ample and were swathed in sheets of antiseptic wool. A copious bandaging with gauze bandages followed, no regard being paid to the classical types so carefully taught and so prettily applied of the old stiff calico ones then in vogue.

In London we *could* bandage; it was an art that every dresser acquired. 'Parallel and equidistant' was the rule for the encircling turns, the thing aimed at being 'to walk upstairs' with the first two fingers upon the steps of a properly bandaged part. There were spicas and capitella, and many other types; whited sepulchres when one thinks of the microbes imprisoned beneath, but the finished product looked excellent, and dresser and patient were pleased.

With the flexible gauze bandage all this was disregarded. It was a 'go as you please', straining the bandage where necessary or halting it with safety-pins when this was impossible, and starting again; but it was efficient and comfortable, and that was the only thing that mattered.

After a dressing was finished he would turn to the patient with his charming smile, and ask: 'Now are you quite comfortable?'

William Ernest Henley *Letter to Harry Nichols,*
December 1873

Reserved Ward B.
Royal Infirmary
Edinburgh.
16/12/73,

Fiend!

I have been for some time minded to write to ye, in spite of the devilishly characteristic silence with which you have darkened my last letter. But I wanted to tell you something good, so I waited. And now it is too late, for the present, to write happy tidings so that I must, if I would write at all, speak of things as they are and (of course!) ought not to be.

I ought to describe my first operation, that you may the better understand the second. There was a long cut across the foot, from ankle to ankle, dividing vessels, tendons and everything, and laying open the affected bone, which in its turn was scooped out (gouge & pliers), so that a large triangular cavity was the result, the apex of which pointed to the toes. This cavity was filled with strips of lint steeped in carbolic oil; changed, first of all, every four hours, then every eight hours, then twice a day, then once a day: the leg itself being bandaged onto a long iron splint, and the foot pulled out so as to expose every part of the internal surface of the cavity to the action of the oil. In this position it was left to granulate (granulations are the most elementary form of tissue: flesh in embryo in fact); the Professor intending, when the whole surface should be completely covered with granulations, to bring the lips of the wound together and leave them to unite and heal. It was this last operation that I expected to have to announce to you; and, of course, I ain't able to do so.

I fully expected, when I was borne to the Theatre, on Sunday last (in a long basket, like poultry!), to return with my foot replaced and fixed up for healing; for Mr. Lister had almost notified as much to me once or twice during the week. When I came to my senses, however, I was in no wise surprized to find that a lot more bone had been removed, and that I was as far from the Second Act as ever. I have seen my foot since then, and I can assure you, Mephisto mine, that the aspect of it is not calculated to put me in spirits, or to give me any higher opinion of my wretched self than the tolerably cynical one I have already.

Nevertheless, I am informed in good authority that I am 'a good case' and that Mr. Lister is confident of being able to to save my foot. He is a great surgeon, my boy! Antiseptic surgery – his theory and practice – will have to fight its way, to fight for life indeed, and it will be long ere it is generally adopted. But already I think I am justified in saying that, next to the use of anaesthetics, it is the most beneficent discovery of the century. Joseph Lister is an Englishman and (whether he save my foot or no) we may rejoice therefore. The conceit of these bloody Scotchmen is something atrocious.

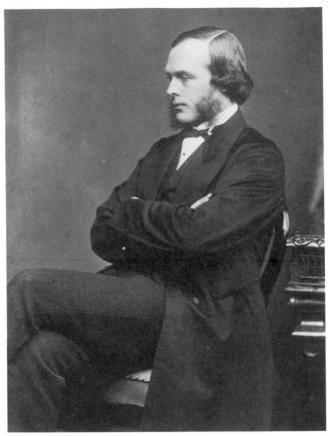

Joseph Lister, aged about 40.

THE CHIEF in *Poems* (1898)

His brow spreads large and placid, and his eye
Is deep and bright, with steady looks that still.
Soft lines of tranquil thought his face fulfill –
His face at once benign and proud and shy.
If envy scout, if ignorance deny,
His faultless patience, his unyielding will,
Beautiful gentleness and splendid skill,
Innumerable gratitudes reply.
His wise, rare smile is sweet with certainties,

And seems in all his patients to compel
Such love and faith as failure cannot quell.
We hold him for another Herakles,
Battling with custom, prejudice, disease,
As once the son of Zeus with Death and Hell.

Here, conventionally, a modern hospital story would end:
both Henley and Mathewson had survived their operations.
But in fact for both of them this was only the first station of their
particular crosses. Margaret was operated on after a month,
and then spent seven months in the hospital; Henley was
operated on within a week of his arrival in Edinburgh, and then
spent twenty months in bed.

Their responses to their enforced stays were true to their
characters. Margaret found solace in religion, and evangelical
work in the wards. For Henley it was an opportunity to catch up
on the education his illness had deprived him of, and to indulge
in more earthly pleasures – in thought.

RECOVERY ON THE WARD

Margaret Mathewson   *Sketch*

I felt anxious to get a few lines written to father by that day's mail as I knew they were anxious regarding me after Dr. Cheyne writing Mr. Barclay. But the difficulty was 'How shall I steady my paper as my left hand is bandaged down and useless at present?' I had put paper for this purpose in a little basket and got the nurse to bring it from Ward 3. I thus got it out, laid it on my chest (as I was down on my back) steadied it with my chin and scrawled about ¾ of a sheet in pencil to father, then scrawled Arthur's usual note telling him the extent of my operation and sent it to him by the nurse.

Letter to her brother Arthur, 25 March 1877

2 Surgical Ward
R In.ʸ
Sunday 25 77

Dear Brother,

I write this to let you know I am a little stronger to night. I continued vomiting till near morning when I ast a teaspoon of brandy and got it and then a drink of lemonade and what lots of ice I have eaten. This morning I took about ½ inch of bread and a little tea and then I got some brandy and ice together and I got free of the vomiting and was able to take some dinner also and a little tea. Dr. Chᶜ has dressed my arm today he says theres no sign of putrification in it.

Professor hasn't been today.

2 Lees's...
R. Inn
Sunday 25 '47

Dear Brother   I write this...

It you know I am a
little stronger to night —
I continue Brandy till —
near morning when I get a
teaspoon of Brandy & ½ a
teaspoon a drink of Momentum.
that ... ice I Momentum
½ to ½ ice I took about ½
this morning I took about ½
inch a teas — a little ...
and then I got some Brandy
& ice together & I got free
of the Vomiting & was able
to take some Momentum also
a little tea   Dr. Ch

... has dressed my every thing
he say there's nothing
putrification in it.
Professor has not been
today.
The child is a little
better but still is considered
dangerous this is very
is not allowed.
Thanks for the
drops & I hope you
will soon get ...
I hope I will be stronger
yours truly
M Mh

The child is a little better but still considered dangerous thus the visitors is not allowed.

Thanks for the drops, and I hope you will soon get in and I hope I will be stronger.

Yours truly
MCM

Margaret's remark about eating in the letter was probably to quell any fears Arthur might have. In the sketch she writes:

I could take no food until the 5th day, as when I saw the nurse bring in the meals I began to vomit. She brought tea to me, but I had to beg of her to take it away as it made me so sick to see any food. On the 5th day she again brought a jug of milk and sais 'Now Maggie you must try one mouthful.'

'No nurse, I really cannot, as I am going to be sick again.'

'Well, I'll leave it here and hope to find some out of it when I come back.'

I thought 'Well I might try one spoonful as I am only vomiting whatever and milk has a tendency of stopping that.' I thus took a little, and waited to see its effects, when I felt the sick feeling wear away and I took some more. Nurse came back: 'Now that's what I like to see.'

'Now nurse will you please infuse me a cup of tea?'

'I will soon do that,' she said laughing. 'You see there's nothing like facing up your difficulties Maggie.'

This is to jump ahead somewhat. Returning to the Sunday evening:

About 7 p.m. I grew very weak and the nurses seemed alarmed I had taken a bad turn. One of them called the Doctor. He came and felt my pulse. 'Dear-o-me nurse, what's this from? What has she been doing?'

'I don't know sir, as I have been off duty this afternoon.'

'Margaret, what have you been doing this afternoon?'

'Nothing, sir, but scrawling a few lines to father.'

93

'What, writing!! However could you write? I do hope you have not attempted to sit up as remember you have to be on your back for a fortnight.'

'No, sir, I did not sit up to do it. I laid the paper here on my chest, steadied it with my chin and wrote with a pencil.'

'Oh, I am so sorry to think of you doing this as first you may lose your eyesight, then it's laid you back a full month, I'm sure.'

'I hope not sir.'

I got better every day after that, but had to lie on my back without turning to either side for a full fortnight which was one of the hardest orders to comply with I got during my eight months there; and I thought if I had to stay anytime in bed I should never get used to it but I did.

Brother Arthur stopped in Edinburgh 2 months. The weather changed to be very wet, and he got worse in health, and thereby laid back 8 or 10 months: but he came to see me every evening during the two months. Also a great many acquaintances came to see me during the time I was there. Thus I generally had as many visitors as any other patient, but I felt very dull when Arthur went home.

William Ernest Henley   *Letters to Harry Nichols*
September 1873

I am tied to a big iron splint and can't move off my back. There is a tremendous gash in my foot but I have suffered – comparatively speaking – little. Try and send me a few shillings, for I am that hard up, and I have such an appetite I don't know what to do. If you could but send me some mutton and pickles! – Peace my soul! –

18 December 1873

. . . I am well enough off for books, especially French books. If you want to know anything about Baudelaire's *Fleurs du Mal* I can tell you that, in my opinion, they are real flowers, no artful *pastiche* of some clever *fleuriste* but genuine flowers, lustrous and metallic of leaf, strange and violent of odour, poison flowers, flowers from the Devil's hot-house perhaps, but real for all that.

19 December 1873

. . . I have read over my letter to you, old man, and find it dull: I suppose you will do the same. I decided on flattering your physiological instincts with a description of the operation and I fear I haven't succeeded as I ought. Perhaps you'll pitch these sheets unread into the drawer, light up that ineffable pipe (for the forty-seventh time) swear at the matches, or the 'bacca, enwrap your manly form in the celebrated blanket – all things to all men – fling yourself on the immortal sofa and curl yourself into one of those wicked sleeps where you dreamed of the mischief you woke to do . . .

17 May 1874

. . . I have read out the Library here: they have nothing to send me now but garbage, or trash, or history. I am in despair. I seldom or never read English: why I don't know, for Spencer or Shakespeare are always at my elbow. Alas! that it should satisfy my conscience to know they *are* there . . .

I am wearying for a little cold mutton and pickles, for a tune on the piano, for a sniff of the smoke and sawdust of a bar, for a taste of Irish 'ot – when shall we?*

---

* Henley had been introduced to the mysteries of 'Irish 'ot' in Margate in 1872:

> . . . Irish whiskey, otherwise Potheen, otherwise Fenian, is a fluid possessed of extraordinary properties. I shall not stop to communicate any other than this: Taken Hot, with Sugar, and a thin shaving of Lemon-peel, it encourages, in him who imbibes, a tendency to stand for many hours over a bar, while it imparts to him an unusual facility of agreeable and audacious speech. I can vouch for this, which is indeed a result of long and patient observation on my part. Miss Crump [the barmaid] is of the same opinion.

My back aches so, I can sit up no more: my romance cost me over three and half hours work this morning, so that I'm tired. If you can suggest any changes, be a good fellow and do so: I am so long away, I know not whether my London lingo is all it should be. I will write again soon.

Lister's attempts to excise tuberculous joints rather than amputate them inevitably meant that his patients had to spend a long time in hospital, much longer than the convalescent periods of other surgeons' cases.

In March 1875, the Board of the Royal Infirmary complained about the number of Lister's long-term patients. In particular they asked him to comment on four patients: John Wright, who had been in hospital for 389 days, Annie McCanna, 567 days, Jane Maid, 696 days and W. E. Henley who had then been in 565 days. All had tuberculosis.

In reply, Lister quoted a Russian surgeon who had found 'although the antiseptic treatment had led to the retention in hospitals of some patients for a very much longer time than was formerly the case (this being commonly caused by persons being kept alive who without antiseptic treatment would have died) yet on the other hand this mode of treatment cures other patients much more quickly . . . and that to so great an extent that the latter effect more than counterbalances the former.'[33]

The Managers had to accept Lister's reply, but were not happy (see p. 136).

William Ernest Henley

VIGIL in *Poems* (1898)

Lived on one's back,
In the long hours of repose
Life is a practical nightmare –
Hideous asleep or awake.

Shoulders and loins
Ache . . . !
Ache, and the mattress,
Run into boulders and hummocks
Glows like a kiln, while the bedclothes –
Tumbling, importunate, daft –
Ramble and roll, and the gas,
Screwed to its lowermost,
An inevitable atom of light,
Haunts, and a stertorous sleeper
Snores me to hate and despair.

All the old time
Surges malignant before me;
Old voices, old kisses, old songs
Blossom derisive about me;
While the new days
Pass me in endless procession:
A pageant of shadows
Silently, leeringly wending
On . . . and still on . . . still on!

Far in the stillness a cat
Languishes loudly. A cinder
Falls, and the shadows
Lurch to the leap of the flame. The next man to me
Turns with a moan; and the snorer,
The drug like a rope at his throat,
Gasps, gurgles, snorts himself free, as the night-nurse,
Noiseless and strange,
Her bull's eye half-lanterned in apron,
(Whispering me, 'Are ye no sleepin' yet?')
Passes, list-slippered and peering,
Round . . . and is gone.

Sleep comes a last –
Sleep full of dreams and misgivings –
Broken with brutal and sordid
Voices and sounds that impose on me,
Ere I can wake to it,
The unnatural, intolerable day.

Margaret Mathewson   *Sketch*

I went to sleep and soon after was awoke by fearful
screams of 'Murder, Murder!!' just outside the window
and we were so frightened by these words on waking it
seemed so dreadful. Nurse Michi came in.

'Oh nurse, who is that outside?'

'It's some drunk man kicking his wife down the
Cowgate. The police will soon be after them and they
can't get over our big walls.'

'Well, that's a blessing, nurse.'

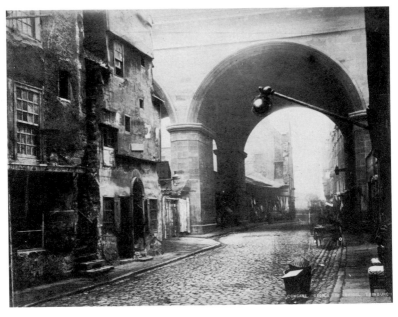

The Cowgate area of Edinburgh, squalid even for
Victorian times.

William Ernest Henley

NOCTURN in *Poems* (1898)

At the barren heart of midnight,
When the shadow shuts and opens
As the loud flames pulse and flutter,
I can hear a cistern leaking.

Dripping, dropping, in a rhythm,
Rough, unequal, half-melodious,
Like the measures aped from nature
In the infancy of music;

Like the buzzing of an insect,
Still, irrational, persistent . . .
I must listen, listen, listen
In a passion of attention;

Till it taps upon my heartstrings,
And my very life goes dripping,
Dropping, dripping, drip-drip-dropping,
In the drip-drop of the cistern.

Margaret Mathewson   *Sketch*

I was almost asleep when the alarm bell rang and instantly
there was an unaccountable noise, all in confusion, people
shouting, some lamenting, some moaning with pain, some
running to and fro, horses prancing about and cabs
coming into the doors etc. I thought this must be some
Railway accident and it was a man that had got run over
and so bruised and crushed at the station, Prof. Lister had
to be sent for. He came but could do nothing for the man
as he was too far gone.

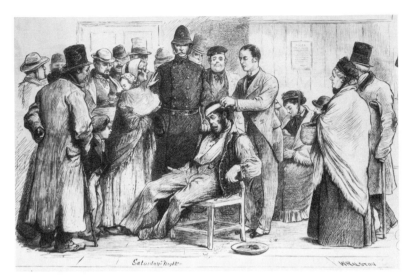

Saturday night in the Casualty Ward. (BBC Hulton Picture Library)

William Ernest Henley

CASUALTY in *Poems* (1898)

As with varnish red and glistening
Dripped his hair; his feet looked rigid;
Raised, he settled stiffly sideways:
You could see his hurts were spinal.

He had fallen from an engine,
And been dragged along the metals.
It was hopeless, and they knew it;
So they covered him, and left him.

As he lay, by fits half-sentient,
Inarticulately moaning,
With his stockinged soles protruded
Stark and awkward from the blankets,

To his bed there came a woman,
Stood and looked and sighed a little,
And departed without speaking,
As himself a few hours after.

In their early days railways were a lethal form of transport. *Punch* and the other magazines of the day listed major smashes weekly. During her eight months in hospital, Margaret recorded two separate incidents. Henley's was a third.

Margaret Mathewson   *Letter to her father, 6 March 1877*

... I have no idea how long they may keep one or how soon I may be out but I like the Infirmary very well as we have every attention paid to us both day and night, theres a big fire and all things strictly clean and tidy all day and plenty of bread tea and all night the fire is blazing and gas burning and a nurse, going among the patients of 2 or 3 rooms but some days there's very bad cases comes in – almost every now and again there's some one carried in, hurled in* or driven in by a cab. And a lot of them is dressed in our ward or room and its awful sights sometimes. I know you would soon run out if you saw them every day as we do and at the very time we are at dinner too, sometimes, but we just sit still and goes on with our dinner and gets used to them things although it's disagreeable, but I always turn my back to them.

Letter to her brother Arthur, 19 July 1877

... I duly received yours of the 12th yesterday and am very glad to see by it you are all in usual and busy with the turnips etc ...

You are thinking my shoulder will be healed over by this time but *it's not healed* up yet and is still discharging a

---

* This is a Shetland expression for 'brought in by wheelbarrow'.

little. For the past fortnight I've only had half a bed and it so hot two in a bed with the bed so small. This last week I had to lie just in any bed who would let me in and I have always had to lie on that person's left side and then my sore arm came to be half over the bed and consequently I was often more tired and weary when I rose than when I lay down. Some nights I'm very tired running out and in all day from 6.30 a.m. to 8.30 p.m. as if you have got 2 fingers and your feet you must give them to the nurses i.e. work. There is new patients crowding in every day but its great nonsense in those who admits them without having room for them. Mary who lay behind the door with the sore foot went away last night apparently incurable as the Dr. told her last week there was a diseased bone still in it and she was to go thro' another operation and then yesterday they told her they would put a water glass on it and try that and she could get away. Her friends were very pressing for her to get away now either cured or not. Sally got a water glass on her knee and she also went away last night, but before they were well away their beds was filled up again and still there's 12 patients in this ward and 16 in No. 3.

Margaret later explains what a water glass is:

... The 'water glass' is made of starch and 60 yds of muslin made into bandages (of 20 yards long); then these bandages wet in the starch; then the leg put into wadding: then a splint over that to keep the leg in the proper position: then the bandages rolled round all. Thus there's no glass at all. This is kept on until pain is felt; then repeated over and over if need be.

Sketch

There was a young woman who came in on Sunday with a 'Docile abscess' below the shoulder blade. She was put to bed at my left side and Marion Forrest was shifted to No. 3. But I had a hope I would profit by it, which indeed I did, as I found her to be an experienced Christian young

102

woman. Her name was Lindsay Matthie. She preferred being called Linna. Half an hour after she lay down, Professor came in, also a lot of students and prepared for an operation, apparently in the ward but I hope not as I dread seeing or hearing anything of this nature and I so weak.

But in a little her bed was drawn across the floor opposite the window for the light. They gave her the chloroform and went on with the operation. I kept the sheet o'er my face for a while and was much affected by knowing what was being done.

After Prof. had gone out and the bed put back I saw the blood on the floor. I grew so weak I almost fainted, and the nurse came and stayed with me a little. It was some days ere I got over the sensation.

William Ernest Henley

THE VISIT in *Cornhill Magazine* (1875)

A many-footed rush resounds without,
Through the long, flagged, deep-vaulted corridor,
And in the Surgeon strides, at least three-score
Of pupils with him – learner, dandy, lout.

He walks as one who is not vexed with doubt;
They straggle after him across the floor,
Silent respectful of his place and lore,
Not always keen for what he is about.

Presenting to contemplative beholders
A curious plump of sentient backs and shoulders,
They group themselves about a certain bed;

A few short words you cannot catch, are said;
Then comes a silence, and your pulses quicken;
And then a crunch of bone and steel – You sicken.

Linna was taken out of the chloroform by dipping a towel in cold water, and slapping her on the face and chest. She got on very well after the operation but then took a bad turn. She got a most violent headache and at the same time consumptive signs were visible, which gave rise to the suggestion of her removal to the Medical House. Linna on hearing this at once said:

'I shall go home and die, not there.'

Professor Stewart from The Medical was called down to examine Linna. He said 'It is consumption, together with a deranged brain, but the patient would be better to stay in "The Surgical" as the change would do more harm than good.'

She was thus left with us, but soon got quite insane; continued so for almost a fortnight, then one morning she awoke with her usual composure, but looked around astonished like. Then her eye resting on me, she smiled, holding out her hand said: 'Good morning, Maggie.'

'Good morning, Linna. I am so glad to see you a little better.'

'Yes, thank God, I am a wee better, but Maggie tell me where they have had me? Not in the medical I hope.'

'No Linna, believe me you have never been from my side but you have been very ill.'

Then Miss Logan came in and went on past us. I said 'Miss Logan, please.'

She turned at once as usual. Pointing to Linna, I said 'Here's Linna, back again.'

Miss Logan grasped Linna's outheld hand and said 'Linna, are your really yourself once more?'

'Yes, I hope so.'

Linna's brothers and sister were in town but her parents were in Kinross. They were sent for and all came by turns to see Linna. But two days after she got worse again (not insane). Her mother and sister were allowed to stop all night as death was seen approaching. She talked such comforting words to her mother and sister assuring them she had a good hope through Jesus of Heaven. She put her arm round her mother's neck and said 'Mother dear, do not cry for me. To the believer in Jesus, death is only a sleep, as Jesus has taken away its terrors. Yea, though I walk through the valley of the shadow of death I will fear no evil: For thou are with me; thy rod and thy staff they comfort me, and it will only be a short time until we shall all meet again. Now Jesus is come and calling for me. Good night all.' And she fell asleep in Jesus about 2 a.m.

I felt Linna's death very much indeed, as she was an experienced exemplary Christian. But our loss was her infinite gain. Linna's remains were not put in the mortuary as usual, but kept in the 'private ward' where she died, and there laid out, superintended by Miss Pringle, the matron. There was a beautiful bouquet of flowers (from a hot house) put on her chest. Her brothers brought a beautiful coffin, which was carried shoulder high to the gate. All of us tried to get the last look of a friend and companion. Some one said 'I wonder who will be next from this ward.'

I said 'Likely I.'

All by turns said 'No perhaps me.'

I said 'Well it's a call to each "me" here. "Be ye also ready, for in such an hour as ye think not, the Son of man cometh."'

Linna's bed was soon filled up again, but with a person very different from Linna.

William Ernest Henley   *Letter to Harry Nichols,*
undated but probably January 1875

. . . How many of us die with our work half done, our lives half lived! Happy they that can write *finis* and then lie down. What is to be for us? –

ANOTHER [Night Picture] in *Cornhill Magainze* (1875)

Round one poor bed is stretched the painted screen
Whose leaves extemporise a decent gloom,
Where Death and Life, as in a private room,
Meet, and arrange the honours of the scene.

The shadows melt into the growing grey;
The gas burns pale. My thoughts are gruesome yet,
But my vague sense of impotent regret
Fades in my pipe's blue tender whorls away.

Before the creaking fire the widow cries,
Huddled and hushed; the fresh young night-nurse dozes;
We talk by fits or think – for in this wise

A gaunt Perhaps itself to us discloses;
And lo, the sun! strong for his new emprise,
All hope and Health, superb with wild mist roses.

Margaret Mathewson   *Sketch*

Next dressing day Prof. dressed me again, then asked me
to let him see how I could move my arm myself. I did so.
He said, 'Well that's very good.' Prof. then had to go again
to London: we heard he was to be home on Tuesday. The
ward was made extra tidy, and a basin of flowers put on
the table to welcome him back.

He came and dressed me, then said, we will now
dispense with the drainage tubes. (This I was thankful to
hear as that was a marked sign of progression.)

It has often been said that Lister invented drainage tubes
under the spur of necessity in the course of a rather important
operation in 1871, unaware that a French surgeon had introduced them in 1859. This is wrong, since in Lister's Glasgow
Ward Books, drainage tubes are referred to in 1865.[34] Be that as
it may, it certainly is true that the use of irritating disinfectants
in large quantities in antiseptic surgery caused wounds to
discharge heavily, and made drainage tubes an indispensable
part of the treatment. Certain schools of surgery went so far as
to pour water continuously over wounds to flush away germs.
Although Lister did not invent the use of the drainage tube in
1871, the story of the operation is none the less a nice one.

Lister had been appointed Surgeon in Ordinary in Scotland to Queen Victoria in 1870. On 3 September 1871, he received a telegram from Balmoral saying that the Queen had developed a large, painful and most undignified abscess in her left armpit.

Lister arrived on 4 September, and decided that an operation was necessary. Queen Victoria noted in her Journal:

> Sir William Jenner explained everything about my arm to him, but he naturally said he could do nothing or give any opinion till he had made an examination. I had to wait nearly half an hour before Mr. Lister and Dr. Marshall appeared! In a few minutes he had ascertained all & went out again with the others. Sir William Jenner returned saying Dr. Lister thought the swelling ought to be cut; he could wait twenty-four hours, but it would be better not. I felt dreadfully nervous, as I bear pain so badly. I shall be given chloroform, but not very much, as I am so far from well otherwise, so I begged the part might be frozen, which was agreed. Sir William Jenner gave me some whiffs of chloroform whilst Mr. Lister froze the place, Dr. Marshall holding my arm. The abscess, which was six inches in diameter, was very quickly cut and I hardly felt anything excepting the last touch, when I was given a little more chloroform. In an instant there was relief. I was then tightly bandaged, and rested on my bed. Quite late saw Beatrice and Alfie for a moment, after Mr. Lister had been in to see me. Felt very shaken and exhausted.[35]

Jenner, the President of the Royal College of Physicians and Physician in Ordinary to the Queen, was given the clerk's job of holding the spray during the operation. Being unused to the job, at one point he gave the Queen a squirt in the eyes; she complained, and he excused himself, saying he was 'only the man who worked the bellows'.

The next day, however, on changing the dressing, Lister found the wound full of pus:

> It occurred to me that in that deep and narrow incision, the lint, instead of serving as a drain, might have acted like

107

a plug, and so reproduced the conditions present before evacuation. Taking a piece of the india-rubber tubing of a Richardson's spray producer that I had used for local anaesthesia at the operation, I cut holes in it and attached knotted silk threads to one end, so improvising a drainage-tube. This I put to steep for the night in a strong watery solution of carbolic acid, and introduced it in place of the lint on changing the dressing next morning. The with-drawal of the lint had been followed by discharge of thick pus as before; but next morning I was rejoiced to find nothing escape unless it were a drop or so of clear serum. This rapidly diminished, and within a week of the opening of the abscess I was able to take leave of my patient, the discharge from the abscess cavity having entirely ceased.[36]

Victoria described the operation as 'a most disagreeable duty most pleasantly performed'; Lister was able, truthfully, to claim to be 'the only man who has ever stuck a knife into the Queen.'

When Queen Victoria agreed to take chloroform to assist her through the birth of one of her children, the publicity did the anaesthetic 'movement' a power of good. Unfortunately, the same did not happen here. While childbearing was a noble and queenly occupation, having an abscess was not, and the operation was not reported until 1908.

Margaret Mathewson   *Sketch*

Professor then said 'Gentlemen, this excision was only made as an experiment. I meant first to amputate the arm but I thought again and again how I could save it, and at last concluded an excision as an experiment and if that did not succeed (as I did not expect it would) then amputation was inevitable. But Providentially, it has been a perfect success and now we will ask her how she can use the joint herself. Will you let me see you can get your finger tips on mine here?' (laying his hand down on the bed at a certain distance from me). I got my finger tips into the palm of his hand.

'Oh, that's very good. Now try and reach mine here' (shifting his hand). I reached it again.

'That's also good. Now can you touch your pillow at your back?'

I got my hand to the top of it. 'Oh, that's excellent. Now try to touch the palm of your hand. Yes all excellent. Now gentlemen, you see how the patient can use it. This arm will be much more useful than wood, or cork, yes, than even a gold one, could we have given her that, instead of this the natural one. And I have no doubt it will yet be as strong as the other one, but it must take some time for that. She has suffered a great deal but patience has her perfect work.'

Prof. told Dr. Roxburgh* (as they went out) to tell me to get up in a day or two and I felt very thankful to God for it, recollecting how many had been called away by death during these 3 months I have been in bed and I the most unlikely spared. Miss Logan came in. I said 'I have got a surprise Miss Logan.'

'What's that?'

'I am told to get up once more.'

'Are you really? Well, I told you lately, you would be getting that surprise some day soon. Now where's your clothes, stockings and stays first, you know.'

'Yes Miss Logan, that used to be the way, but I'm afraid it will yet be some time ere I use my stays as my arm occupies that place.'

'Oh, I forgot.'

'I think my clothes are all here in the drawer.'

'Well, there's not a thing here you require.'

---

* Dr. Roxburgh was Cheyne's replacement as House Surgeon. Margaret wrote:

At the end of 5 weeks, Dr. Cheyne's 6 months as 'House Surgeon' was out, and a Dr. Roxburgh appointed his successor. I was indeed sorry to hear of this change, as I always looked to Dr. Cheyne as a friend. But ere he left he brought Dr. Roxburgh into the ward, and to each bed side and explained each case to him. When they came to mine Dr. Cheyne after explaining the case said, 'Now Dr. will you please treat this patient kindly, as she belongs to the same place as I do.'

'Oh, Yes Dr. I shall' and he invariably did so.

'Oh, Miss Logan, it's all at my boarding in Leith as I sent it down to get washed and ready for me getting up!'

'Well whatever will you do, as you must get up when you are told, but not sooner.'

'I will go on beggary.'

(Miss Logan thought this a fine lark.) Turning round she said 'Ladies, here's a fellow patient told to get up and now all her things are away in Leith – 3 miles off! Whatever will she do? (all laughing). She says she will go on beggary. Do you think she will be a good beggar?'

'Yes, here's my stockings,' said several at once.

Mary Ann Sands said 'Maggie just take my clothes as it is all here together and use it until you get your own.'

'I am much obliged to you all for your kindness.'

Most of them in No. 2 said they hoped I could come and sit down at their bedside. Mary Ann said: 'No Maggie you must come to me first mind.'

'I'm afraid I will have to learn to walk again first, and that will amuse you all for this day. But after that, if spared, I hope to come to you all and have a chat about our Johns.'

Miss Logan dressed me, and I had to learn to walk, sure enough I was so weak, and my feet so sore. I had to rest several times. After sitting a little at the fire I almost fainted; but Miss Logan was with me and got some cold water, then a teaspoon of wine and got me better in a little. A little later Mary Ann asked me to try and come over to her bedside.

I was getting very well acquaint with the patients, but Mary Ann Sands I observed was more sober, sensible and respectable looking than most of those there, and we got to be good friends. She had abscesses in the breast and had two operations and stood it very well. She had been out walking about a week, was to get home the next week when her father came from Stirling and had her out for a drive. While out she got a strange pain below the shoulder blade and her father turned at once for the Infirmary. She was examined and it was found to be a Docile abscess commencing. And ere the other week came round, Mary Ann had got another operation and had become a patient in No. 2.

'I'm afraid I can't walk to you.'

'Take it by stages.'

I got over and sat down. Then she began to cry and said 'Oh Maggie'.

'Yes, I know. After being 5 long weary months in bed, and then to be told to get up and that you could get home next week, and then to be put through another operation instead is indeed a great disappointment. But Mary Ann, believe me, it is for some good end. God never afflicts us nor any person willingly. He tries one sort of affliction and if that does not help us to turn unto him, God is pleased sometimes to repeat our afflictions again and again as he works by means to draw our hearts out after himself.'

'I do envy you on a something you seem to possess thro' religion which seems to guide your conversation and daily life. And now you must please to tell me all about it so as I can get it and die happy as I feel sure I shall never get up again.'

'Well! I have got a message for you and it is this. "Though your sins be as scarlet, they shall be as white as snow; though they be red like crimson they shall be as wool!" Well Mary Ann you have on this scarlet flannel jacket. Do you ever think you could ever wash this jacket white?'

'No. I could never do that.'

'Well, what can make them this white? The blood of Jesus Christ, his son, cleanseth us from all sin, Mary Ann, not this sin or that sin but all sin.'

'But Maggie, tell me something to tell Satan as I feel him tempting me not to believe you.'

'Just tell him Mary Ann that the blood of Jesus Christ his son, cleanseth us from all sin, and keep telling him that verse whatever he tells you and he must soon leave you and Jesus will take his place . . .'

Next morning when we awoke she called over: 'Oh, Maggie, I never before had such a night as Satan tempted me so, but I just kept telling him "The blood of Jesus Christ, his Son, cleanseth us from all sin." He then shew me my sins in alphabetical order and it was such a sheet reaching to the very heavens and he asked me if that was not too many to be forgiven. Oh Maggie, I felt ashamed and was about giving up trying any longer when instantly the words came to my help. "The blood of Jesus Christ cleanseth from all sin" and I saw Jesus on the cross, yes the very nails in his hands and feet, Maggie, and the blood tipping from the fingers and Oh, the look of extreme suffering on his face. But he looked on me and smiled saying "I suffer this for thee" and I fell at the foot of the cross and saw his precious blood trickling down on my sheet of sin and instantly I saw it all wiped out, and Jesus Christ standing between eternal death and my soul.'

'Well I must interrupt you and say we can go no further until we have first thanked our heavenly Father for this.' I was very much excited by Mary Ann's confession I grew so weak and felt faintish, the cold sweat running down my forehead.

'Maggie what is wrong with you?'

'Mary Ann, it touches me so to see that I have been used by God to carry a message of salvation to a sinner. Believe me it is for some good end you were disappointed of getting home and will become a blessing and cause you thankfulness instead of regret.'

'Yes, Maggie, it is the very best I have met with since I came here and do you know that long before I got badly at home I wished I might get badly and have to go to this Infirmary as I felt I had to get some great thing or do some great thing in this house!'

Mary Ann Sands died while I was at the convalescent. But I saw her the day previous to her death and she was resting peacefully on Christ's finished work and thus had a bright hope of heaven. But I found another companion in religion in the same ward, viz. Agnes Templeton.

William Ernest Henley

SUICIDE in *Poems* (1898)

Staring corpselike at the ceiling,
See his harsh, unrazored features,
Ghastly brown against the pillow,
And his throat – so strangely bandaged!

Lack of work and lack of victuals,
A debauch of smuggled whisky,
And his children in the workshouse
Made the world so black a riddle.

That he plunged for a solution;
And, although his knife was edgeless;
He was sinking fast towards one,
When they came, and found, and saved him.

In his broad face, tanned and bloodless,
White and wild his eyeballs glisten;
And his smile, occult and tragic,
Yet so slavish, makes you shudder!

Margaret Mathewson   *Sketch*

There was a patient in No. 3 with a twisted elbow joint.
She was put to bed and her arm tied round with straps,
then a cord tied into the straps and put over a bit of cord
about a foot high which was fixed on the foot of the bed
and then 7 lb of sand put into a little bag and hung on the
cord out side of the foot of the bed near the floor. This 7 lb
of sand was on the cord a few days then 7 lb more was
added; the 14 lb was on a few days, then 7 lb was again
added. Prof. was at London at the time and Dr. Chiene of
Edinburgh was acting Professor instead.* He thus made
the operation, viz. 'excised' the elbow joint. She continued
very weak during the evening and seemed to get worse as
the evening wore on. Dr. Cheyne came and took her pulse
every half hour, and a special nurse was set at her bedside.
Dr. Cheyne came with a medicine glass full of morphia
and offered to her. She was very against taking it. He
pressed on her to take it, and it would make her better. She
did so after some persuasion. She was very ill all night and
next day restless and anxious, looking as if she was

---

* 'John Chiene', writes Leeson in *Lister as I Knew Him,* 'took charge of the ward
during the Professor's absence, and it was strange the difference it made.
There was no "Mr." then, we were a team working comfortably together and
happily at our ease (see p. 51). We asked questions, discussed cases, had
even an occasional joke and sometimes a little tale; but immediately the
Professor appeared we were on parade duty.'

frightened she was about to die. She said, 'Why do they make us eat ice?'

'I have heard it said that ice helps the wounds on, as it keeps down inflamation.'

'That's singular but I believe I am not going to get better, but have come here to die very likely.'

'Oh, no, I think you are looking better than you were yesterday.'

'I do not feel any better.'

'Well, that is doubtless owing to the chloroform. Its effects will stay with you some time after you are got over the operation. But I hope if you do not get better that you will get home to heaven where there's no more pain.'

'Oh, Yes. Father will plead for me.'

'You mean Father "Really" as you call him.'

'Yes.'

'Well I do not wish to say anything against any creed but, believe me, the priest cannot save your never dying soul nor bring you absolution (or forgiveness). Jesus is a priest for every sinner, he is the real priest, who has pleaded and is pleading for us at this moment, and we can tell him much better than we can tell any other person about our sins, and whatever we have to tease us. And do you know he is here listening to us at this moment.'

She looked round then said, 'You do talk strange, Margaret, but have you ever been a "Catholic" as you seem to know all about us so well?'

'No indeed I have never been, and I would never be one, but I have lived with Roman Catholic people, and have read about them and their ceremonies. Jesus is in heaven there to speak for us, and we can tell him everything and he tells his Father, and thus there is no use for a priest between Jesus and you at all, as that only makes God angry and heaps sin on your own soul.'

'Well I could never talk to God myself as he is so good and grand and far above me.'

'I must tell you that you must talk to him yourself, either by prayer now or at the judgement bar after Death.'

'Well I will speak to father about it.'

'No just try and speak to Jesus once without the priest.'

'No, No I could not.'

'Well the priest cannot do anything for you whatever, and if you go on trusting him to make it all right for you

114

with God you will never get to heaven. Believe me I tell you the truth.'

Next day she was better in health and over the idea she was dying and still trusted to her father the priest. She got on well, and was dismissed 'cured' after a time.

William Ernest Henley

A VISITOR in *Cornhill Magazine* (1875)

Her little face is like a walnut shell
With wrinkling lines; her soft white hair adorns
Her either brow in quaint straight curls, like horns,
And all about her clings an old sweet smell.

She wears prim stuffs and puritanic shawls,
Her bonnets might have well been born on her.
Can you conceive a fairy godmother
Devoted to conventicles and calls?

In snow or shine, from bed to bed she runs,
Her mittened hands that always give, or pray,
Bearing a sheaf of tracts, a bag of buns:

All twinkling smiles and texts and pious tales,
A wee old maid that sweeps the Bridegroom's way,
Strong in a cheerful trust that never fails.

Margaret Mathewson   *Sketch*

There was a child of 3 years of age who had a painful disease, and he was put in No. 3 with us, as he required special attention and the nurse at that time could not always be with him but one of us could. It was very sad to see his suffering at times. I often took him on my knee and told him little stories. He thus clung more to me than the

115

others. He got two operations one after the other and stood it very well. He then was to get a third (as he could not stand it all at once). That day his mother came to see him but she had to wait until the afternoon. She was put into No. 1 where I had gone to write some letters as it was so quiet. She asked me if I was a nurse or a patient. 'I am a patient Ma'am.'

'Do you know little Alex.' We spoke about him a little then we heard the doctor go upstairs with him to The Theatre and Alex crying 'Fae you go with me now?'

'Only upstairs, be a good boy.'

At this his mother burst out and cried and then came over to me, laying her hand on my shoulder. I said 'Have you any objections to a few words of prayer.'

'No indeed, I am only sorry I hear too little of that.'

We knelt down and she engaged in prayer, commending her darling boy to God's infinite care and disposal. We both rose up refreshed and I felt she was no stranger to prayer. She stopped all night and sat at Alex's bedside and all next day and the other evening he died. I did feel sorry for his mother, but I knew she was not one of those who did not have God for her friend. Thus I doubt not she took it from His hand who does all things well.

William Ernest Henley

CHILDREN: PRIVATE WARD in *Poems* (1898)

Here in this dim, dull, double-bedded room,
I play the father to a brace of boys,
Ailing but apt for every sort of noise,
Bedfast but brilliant yet with health and bloom.
Roden, the Irishman is 'sieven past',
Blue-eyed, snub-nosed, chubby and fair of face.
Willie's but six, and seems to like the place,
A cheerful little collier to the last.
They eat, and laugh, and sing, and fight, all day;
All night they sleep like dormice. See them play
At Operations: – Roden, the Professor,
Saws, lectures, takes the artery up, and ties;

116

Willie, self-chloroformed, with half-shut eyes,
Holding the limb and moaning – Case and Dresser.

This is Roden Shields, who appeared on p. 45. Here is his description of Henley:

> I cannot remember meeting him for the first time; all I remember is that he lay in one bed and I, with Willie Morrison, lay in the other. He had a plenitude of sandy hair, which, with his rather large front teeth, gave him a fierce aspect. But I had no fear of Henley; we were comrades – he twenty-seven, we six and seven.
>
> I used to be very curious as to his writing so much, and asked him whom he wrote to. He told me his grandmother.

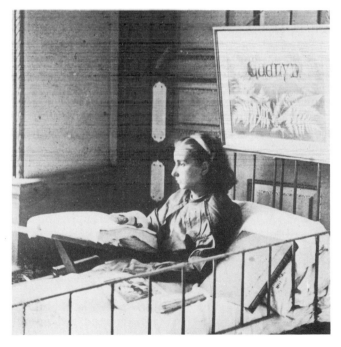

A child in a Victorian hospital. (BBC Hulton Picture Library)

Which reply I thought satisfactory, and considered him an exemplary grandson.

Henley was very kind to us, telling us stories and singing droll ditties, many of them, I believe, original.[37]

Margaret Mathewson   *Sketch*

There was a patient in No. 3 who had a very sore leg from Varicose veins. After trying several sorts of treatment Prof. Lister said, 'There seems to be only one experiment more I would try with this patient, and that is if I could get a bit of live skin off a living person (which I suppose I will not get) I would graft it into the sore on the patient's leg and I believe it would then heal.'

One of the students, a Mr. Peddie, spoke and said, 'Please sir, here's my leg to take it from.' (All in astonishment).

Prof. said 'Are you in earnest, Mr. Peddie?'

'Yes sir, I mean what I say.'

'Thank you kindly, Mr. Peddie. Well then you must go through your operation.'

'Yes sir.'

'Then we will repair to the Theatre, gentlemen.'

All went out and soon returned, and Mr. Peddie was sent home in a cab. Prof. then grafted it into Miss Reid's leg and it got on well every day and did heal, and she was dismissed. Mr. Peddie was off duty for a few days, then came back to shew greater sympathy, as the day following there was a bad railway accident that came in, and the man had lost so much blood that Prof. said, 'He must die unless I could get live blood into his veins.'

Mr. Peddie again said 'Please sir here's my arm.' (!!Pulling up his sleeve).

'Thank you Mr. Peddie it is certainly kind of you to do this, as well as sympathetic.'

Prof. took a bleeding cup off the table, lanced his arm and took the quantity he required, bandaged up Mr. Peddie's arm, then ordered a cab, told the cabman to convert it into an open carriage and drive this gentleman home. Prof. then took the bleeding cup, put the blood little

118

by little into a silver tube about the length of a darning needle also pointed, jagged this tube over the dying man's heart, chest and arms, thus instilling the blood into his veins. He got better every day and was soon dismissed cured.

The two operations described here reveal Lister's (and medicine's) ignorance of immunology.

There was no chance that the skin graft could work: a transplant taken from another person, chosen at random is certain to be rejected. Only now, in the 1980s, are the mechanics of transplantations being successfully worked out. Lister's *failure* was masked by the fact that the immunological system takes a long time to reject a *skin* graft – long enough for the patient, Miss Reid in this case, to appear to be in a stable condition and for her to be dismissed 'cured', so that her bed could be made free for a more pressing case.

Lister was not, quite, pioneering grafting. In the eighteenth century John Hunter had tried animal transplants – of testes and ovaries on cocks and hens – and thought them successful. Others had tried the grafts on people, and succeeded with homo-grafting, a pinch of skin from an undamaged area being applied to a damaged area, such as a burn. From about 1870, with their new-found antiseptic confidence, many surgeons tried the operation.[38]

The blood transfusion, though not so certain to fail, was actually far more dangerous. Given that both the donor and recipient were of the common blood groups, the chance of a mismatch was about 75 per cent. In that event the patient should certainly have been killed. He was probably saved by the extremely inefficient method Lister used to perform the operation: pouring the blood down a narrow tube stuck at various points about the patient's body. There would have been very little 'head' of gravitational pressure to drive the blood in, always providing that Lister had successfully placed his darning needle into a vein, and the clotting of the blood in the tube would have further impeded its flow. It is therefore probable that only a small amount of blood would have been transfused, and if the patient *did* get better, it was from his own natural recuperative powers.

Again, this was not a new operation. Transfusions had been tried in the 1660s, soon after Harvey's work on the circulation of blood. The Frenchman, Jean Baptiste Denis, poured the blood of sheep and calves into his human patients. His first two patients 'recovered', his next two died. The widow of the last sued Denis, but it was proved that she had given her husband arsenic, which weakened her case somewhat. None the less, all this *brouhaha* persuaded surgeons to avoid the operation until the nineteenth century.

The sixth of Lister's celebrated Glasgow compound fracture cases, John Campbell, brought in with a broken thigh after a large rock had fallen on him in the quarry where he worked, had been offered a blood transfusion. Infection had set in three weeks after the antiseptic operation. Lister had then battled on for four months, until a splinter of bone left behind from the original fracture eroded into an artery. At that point Lister offered him a transfusion – it is not known of whose blood. The dying Campbell refused it.

William Ernest Henley

A STUDENT in *Cornhill Magazine* (1875)

A little black man, admirably neat,
Extremely 'gentleman' from head to foot,
All glossy hat, white shirt, and shiny boot,
Good links and chain, and kerchief smelling sweet.

He soaks his hair in water till the curl
Peculiar to his race will smooth away,
And visits his moustaches day by day,
Though yet, in this respect, a very girl.

His traits? – resentful and suspicious vanity,
Showy dexterity, logical humanity,
Thin brilliance, commonplace intelligence:

And, over all, unquenchable, immense,
Alert to smile and bow, to watch and wait,
An egotism making these things great.

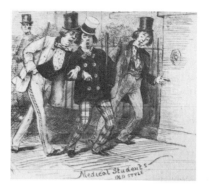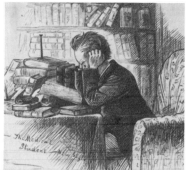

Medical students, old style and new style. As medicine changed so did the calibre of the students it attracted. (BBC Hulton Picture Library)

Margaret Mathewson   *Letter of spring 1877*

. . . There was a girl got a serious operation yesterday and is getting on very well. She's in here. It was a large lump across her throat, falling down on her chest rather. They were about 3 hours over it and when she came down Professor L^r came and sat down at her bedside over ¼ of an hour slapping her on the side of the head with a wet handkerchief, and putting brandy about her lips and then she wakened. He stayed with her a little longer trying to get her to speak, but she wouldn't. He called again and again:

'Jessie, how are you?'
No, she wouldn't speak, but she's all right now . . .

John Rudd Leeson   *Lister as I Knew Him*

No trained hospital porter in brown holland overall with india-rubber tyred trolley waited to take the patient to the ward; the dressers formed up, placed the patient on a simple stretcher and carried him as best they could up the long flight of stairs; any serious case Lister invariably accompanied. Arrived in the ward he would direct the movements for lifting the patient, always insisting that the stretcher must be placed at the foot and not at the side of the bed, as seems one of the ineradicable errors of human nature. When three pairs of arms were under the body the word was given, Lister himself taking the head; he then arranged the sand-bags and hot-water bottles, accompanied by invariable warnings of the necessity of their being covered by flannel, and how patients recovering from anaesthesia had been burnt if this was omitted. Finally, with almost womanly care he would replace the bed-clothes, and see that all was snug and comfortable, and as soon as the patient articulated a word would say that all anaesthetic danger was over.

CONVALESCENCE

Margaret Mathewson *Sketch*

A few weeks after this Miss Logan came and said
'Margaret, you and others are ordered out to the
"Convalescent hospital", and here's your cards which
you have to go up stairs to the top where you will see
Dr. Chiene who is the Dr. for the "convalescent". And if
he rejects you on account of so many there we are not loth
of you yet here.'

'Thank you Miss Logan.'

Four of us went upstairs (6 flight). I sat down quite tired
so I had never been up more than 12 steps since I was out
of bed; and I felt so weak much more than I really believed
I was. Thus I hoped all would be admitted but I for some
time yet. But to my dismay none were admitted, but I.
I was so sorry as I dreaded the strong country air. I came
down from seeing Dr. Chiene and lay down on my bed.
Miss Logan came in 'Well, who has passed their
examination?'

'None but I, Miss Logan.'

'Margaret, you just have half an hour for dinner and to
pack your things.'

'I shall never be in time then.'

'Oh, I think you will. Hurry up, and get ready for off.
And the cabs go from the Medical House Door.'

The Convalescent House of the Royal Infirmary had been
opened in 1867 at Corstorphine, two miles west of Edinburgh.
Though now part of Edinburgh's urban sprawl, it was then a
pleasant rural village, surrounded by fields, and with a splendid
view of the Pentland Hills, from where, no doubt, strong country
air would waft.

Margaret Mathewson *Sketch*

I was in time enough for the cabs. Each cab took four patients and charged the Infirmary 10/–. We left about 2 p.m. I enjoyed the drive very much but felt the change of air as we passed through the town into the country. It was about 4 miles from the Infirmary.

At 5 p.m. the tea bell rung and all the men patients went into the dining hall. At 5.30 our bell rung and we all went into the same room, the men having gone out. There were 22 of us at tea and 2 nurses to wait on us. At 8 p.m. supper came, and the men. Then at 8.30 p.m. we went and had nice porridge and milk. Then all went to bed. The whole 22 of us slept in one room. It seemed so nice all to be together, and yet here we are thrown together more than ever we were at the Infirmary as here are patients from all the different apartments in the Infirmary, Medical with all its diversities of disease, Erysipelas, Eye-wards, Fever house and Surgical, sitting together sleeping and walking, which calls for more caution than formerly.

The scenery there was very beautiful and strong bracing air. Inside of the wall was a space of about ½ an acre. First, inside of the gate was Mr. Gavine's house (the gardner), then a row of tall trees along the wall, then a gravel walk (round the enclosure) and rests for the patients: then flowers along one side of the walk; then trees again; then flowers; then green grass; then a wire fence enclosing a square plot of grass; and 12 sheep on it; above which stood the house, those trees and walks going twice round the house. We could see about 4 miles east and west and 5 north. There were also the 'Caledonian' and 'North British' railway lines, and trains day and night, and farmers working in the fields, and the beautiful corn, potatoes, turnips, rye-grass, clover, etc. ripening for reaping. And this itself was a feast to the eye after being shut up in the Infirmary so many months. There was every accommodation in the Convalescent House. There was a sitting ward for the men patients. Overhead was their sleeping ward, dressing room, bath room, and nurses' room. Then were some private patients' rooms; then our bathroom, and nurses' room, our sleeping room and dressing room, below which was our sitting ward. Down the centre was a long table piled up with books for our use.

124

Around were 4 sofas, 6 chairs, 4 long rests and seats, 2 fireplaces, 2 side tables and self-containing writing desk.

Next our ward was Mr. Wilson's room (the overseer), the store rooms, the surgery, the study, the matron's visiting room, then again the general dining hall where I began.

We had coffee bread and butter for breakfast. I always bought a tumbler of new milk and a biscuit at 12 noon for lunch. This I felt doing me much good. Dinner at 1 p.m. We had a change of dinner every day as follows:

Monday, barley soup, thickened with cabbage and cold beef and bread after.

Tuesday, rice soup and cabbage, boiled beef and bread.

Wednesday, potatoes and Irish stew, rice and milk.

Thursday, boiled meat and bread, also barley broth.

Friday, potatoes and hash, also rice and milk.

Saturday, rice soup thickened with leeks, cold meat and bread.

Sunday, roast meat (cold) and bread, also barley broth.

William Ernest Henley   *Letter to Harry Nichols,*
17 May 1874

Now for myself; I need not say I am excessively poor still less need have I to declare myself excessively dull. If it were not for sounds of feline ecstasy in the corridors at night and amorous cawings and twitterings from the crows and sparrows in the quad, I should hardly guess it was May. *I* don't feel like it at all. I have no will to read, and less to write; the songs and sonnets I write occasionally are almost Baudelairian in their bitter fixity of ennui: I have no longings nor illusions; my foot is slowly getting well; at all events it is absolutely painless; but tho' I look excellent well (the women here find me very handsome!) I am anything but satisfied with myself. What I shall be fit for when I get the bullet goodness only knows.

I have been degraded to the ground floor since last I wrote: *autres pays, autres moeurs.* It is a small misshapen room, low-ceiled and flag-floored and the walls are a dirty buff-brown. There are two beds in it, two chairs, two or three worn-out rickety tables and stools; an illumination and a sheaf of hymns hang on the plaster; the sun never shines into it farther than the extreme edge of my bed – in fact it never looks cheery save in the light that gladdens everything however dull and dreary inherently, the pleasant, intelligent blaze of a good hearty FIRE.

I am close to the window and through it I can see the grass-plat in the quad, the sweet sun shining on the daisies and dandelions, chasing the shadows slowly from point to point, along the walls and windows, and flashing on the skylights, like the amiable tyrant he is: I can see the quick, bright sparrows fighting over the crumbs I throw them, the corpulent crows wandering about, breast-high in the grass after belated worms, the hospital terrier, a jolly, ugly lively kindly dog, with the most intelligent tail I ever saw, larking with his friends, barking at the birds and flying (in fun) after the cats who come to sun themselves and snooze on the window-sills after their nocturnal philanderings. I can also see the whole body of nurses and probationers go to dinner and tea, and return, singly and in squads: but this a negative advantage, because of Miss Webb.

Miss Webb is young and fair and English with the sort of skin you like to fancy you are kissing. She is short and would be very well built if she were not *quite* so stout. Her walk is provocative and irritating in the extreme: from her footfall, you can tell that the other end of her leg is satisfactorily heavy also. Miss Webb is the plague of my life; I have made all sorts of attempts to get acquainted with her; if she came once, I say, twisting my moustache, she would certainly come again. – But she won't come once; and this is why I say to myself, with a sigh: 'Oh, Miss Webb!'; why I dream of her in all sorts of improper conjunctures; why I confess I would give all I am worth in this world, my artificial leg included, once with my lips to divide those beautiful breasts, once with my body to open those adorable legs, once with my etc. etc. etc. – Oh, Miss Webb! –

I am resolved to write her some verses in my best, most exquisite vein – epileptic anapaests, sonorous iambics, tinkling trochees – declare my passion, or bust in the attempts. If I only had another leg! – Nick, old pal, there was a real-un lost to the world, when I was spoiled; I regret it, for the sake of all the women on earth.

There she frisks across the quad – adorable wagtail, –
Alas she's gone. Oh, Miss Webb!

ANTEROTICS in *Poems* (1898)

Laughs the happy April morn
Thro' my grimy, little window,
And a shaft of sunshine pushes
Thro' the shadows in the square.

Dogs are tracing thro' the grass,
Crows are cawing round the chimneys,
In and out among the washing
Goes the West at hide-and-seek.

Loud and cheerful clangs the bell,
Here the nurses troop to breakfast.
Handsome, ugly, all are women . . .
O, the Spring – the Spring – the Spring!

Here are the details about Miss Webb, originally written
in a beautiful longhand, from the hospital's records.

Name: Louisa Webb.

Description: Aged 23, single, had been helping a little
in a children's hospital. Recommended by
the Sister-in-Charge of St. Lucy's Hospital,
Gloucester.

**Particulars
of Training:** She was ill nearly two months of the ten she
was here. One month was spent in Medical
wards and seven in Surgical.

Remarks: A good nurse, bright clever and kind. She
gained Dr. Crooms 1st Prize in July 1874.
Her ill health compelled her to leave at the
end of ten months and it was not judged
safe for her to return.

Situations: After leaving us in Oct. 1874 Private
nursing in Brighton and South of England.
Afterwards went to S. Africa.

Margaret Mathewson   *Sketch*

At the infirmary there was a concert for the especial
benefit of the patients to keep their spirits up. This was
every Wednesday during the summer months in the
evening from 7 pm to 8 pm and a piano was hired for a
guinea an hour, and by most patients was very much
appreciated but by others, and myself, quite repugnant.
I was thus very sorry to find a 'concert' also at the
convalescent.

I went twice to it with reluctance, then resolved that I
should stay back unless it was really the 'Rules' which it
cannot be or it evidently would be on the list. All went but
myself, I began reading a religious book. In a little our
nurse came and said in a commanding angry tone. 'Why
are you not at the concert?'

'Because I don't choose to go nurse.'

'Well, it's the rules, *all* to go.'

'Then I humbly beg your pardon. But why then is it not
in the list there? Why should I be compelled to go to any
such place when I can't enjoy it and could employ my time
much better.'

'Well, Margaret, I must now confess, it is not the rules
to compel any person. It is to their option. And now I will
keep you company for a little if you don't object.'

'I will be glad of your company nurse.'

William Ernest Henley

INTERLUDE in *Poems* (1898)

O, the fun, the fun and frolic
That *The Wind that Shakes the Barley*
Scatters through a penny-whistle
Tickled with artistic fingers!

Kate the scrubber (forty summers,
Stout but sportive) treads a measure,
Grinning, in herself a ballet,
Fixed as fate upon her audience.

128

Stumps are shaking, crutch-supported;
Splinted fingers tap the rhythm;
And a head all helmed with plasters
Wags a measured approbation.

Of their mattress-life oblivious,
All the patients, brisk and cheerful,
Are encouraging the dancer,
And applauding the musician.

Dim the gas-lights in the output
Of so many ardent smokers,
Full of shadow lurch the corners,
And the doctor peeps and passes.

There are, maybe some suspicions
Of an alcoholic presence . . .
'Tak' a sup of this, my wumman!' . . .
New Year comes but once a twelvemonth.

Letter to Harry Nichols, 8 December 1874

> I've had one or two letters from Leslie Stephen, Editor of
> the *Cornhill* (whose book on 'True thinking and plain
> speaking' you ought to read) who is coming to Edinburgh
> in February and proposes to visit me.

Leslie Stephen came to Edinburgh to give a lecture on the
Alps. He wrote to his wife:

> . . . I had an interesting visit to my poor contributor. He is
> a miserable cripple in the Infirmary, who has lost one foot
> and is likely to lose another – or rather hopes just to save it,
> and has a crippled hand besides. He has been 18 months
> laid up here and in that time has taught himself Spanish,
> Italian and German, and he writes poems of the
> Swinburne kind, and reads such books as he can get hold
> of. I have taken one of his poems for the *Cornhill*. I went to
> see Stevenson this morning, Colvin's friend, and told him
> about this poor creature, and am going to take him there

this afternoon. He will be able to lend him books and perhaps to read his MSS. and be otherwise useful. So I hope that my coming to Edinburgh will have done good to one living creature.[39]

Robert Louis Stevenson to Mrs Sitwell (later Lady Colvin)

Yesterday Leslie Stephen, who was down here to lecture, called on me and took me up to see a poor fellow, a sort of poet who writes for him, and who has been eighteen

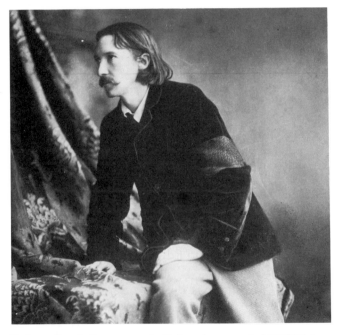

Robert Louis Stevenson in Bohemian mood. (BBC Hulton Picture Library)

months in our infirmary and may be, for all I know, eighteen months more. It was very sad to see him there, in a little room with two beds, and a couple of sick children in the other bed; a girl came in to visit the children and played dominoes on the counterpane with them. The gas flared and crackled, the fire burned in a dull, economical way: Stephen and I sat in a couple of chairs and the poor fellow sat up in his bed with his hair and beard all tangled and talked as cheerfully as if he had been in a King's palace, or the great King's palace of the blue air. He has taught himself two languages since he has been lying there. I shall try to be of use to him. [40]

William Ernest Henley

APPARITION in *Poems* (1898)

Thin-legged, thin-chested, slight unspeakably,
Neat-footed and weak-fingered: in his face –
Lean, large-boned, curved of beak, and touched with race,
Bold-lipped, rich-tinted, mutable as the sea,
The brown eyes radiant with vivacity –
There shines a brilliant and romantic grace,
A spirit intense and rare, with trace on trace
Of passion and impudence and energy.
Valiant in velvet, light in ragged luck,
Most vain, most generous, sternly critical,
Buffoon and poet, lover and sensualist:
A deal of Ariel, just a streak of Puck,
Much Antony, of Hamlet most of all,
And something of the Shorter-Catechist.

Robert Louis Stevenson to Mrs Sitwell, April 1875

My afternoons have been so pleasantly occupied – taking Henley drives. I had a business to carry him down the long stair, and more of a business to get him up again, but while he was in the carriage it was splendid. It is now just the top of spring with us. The whole country is mad with green. To see the cherry-blossoms bitten out upon the black firs, and the black firs bitten out of the blue sky, was a sight to set before a king. You may imagine what it was to a man who had been eighteen months in a hospital ward. The look of his face was a wine to me. [41]

William Ernest Henley

PASTORAL in *Poems* (1898)

It's the Spring.
Earth has conceived, and her bosom,
Teeming with summer, is glad.

Vistas of change and adventure,
Thro' the green land
The grey roads go beckoning and winding,
Peopled with wains, and melodious
With harness-bells jangling:
Jangling and twangling rough rhythms
To the slow march of the stately, great horses
Whistled and shouted along.

White fleets of cloud,
Argosies heavy with fruitfulness,
Sail the blue peacefully. Green flame the hedgerows.
Blackbirds are bugling, and white in wet winds
Sway the tall poplars.
Pageants of colour and fragrance,
Pass the sweet meadows, and viewless
Walks the mild spirit of May,
Visibly blessing the world.

O, the brilliance of blossoming orchards!
O, the savour and thrill of the woods,
When their leafage is stirred
By the flight of the Angel of Rain!
Loud lows the steer; in the fallows
Rooks are alert; and the brooks
Gurgle and tinkle and trill. Thro' the gloamings,
Under the rare, shy stars,
Boy and girl wander   .
Dreaming in darkness and dew.

It's the Spring.
A sprightliness feeble and squalid
Wakes in the ward, and I sicken,
Impotent, winter at heart.

I had been a week at the Convalescent when we heard
Professor Lister had got the Professor's place at St.
Thomas's Hospital London and that he was to be at the
Infirmary for his last time on Wednesday. I asked the
matron for a pass and explained the reason as it was not
my dressing day. I went and Prof. dressed my arm then
said:–

'Gentlemen, I have great pleasure in seeing this case
today and I see a marked progress from when I saw it last.
What a useful experiment this is. It was really as singular
a case as I have had for some years. And to add to it's
singularity, the same day I got this, I also got a man's
shoulder and I tried another experiment with it, but it has
not been so successful as this. I have no doubt of this being
a useful arm yet. In fact it is of use already, as I came
accidently into the ward one day and got her knitting a
stocking to my glad surprise. Let me see how you can use
the arm now. Move it in every direction you can. Now
Gentlemen is not that good of an excised joint? Now
squeeze my hand. That's good. Now this gentleman's.
Yes, really good and I have no doubt it's of use already.'

Lister made frequent trips to London. Margaret records
three disappearances: one in March, a second in early April (he
stayed away for several weeks then) and a third in early May.

Lister had, in fact, long wanted to return to London – his
home town, and where most of the very close Lister family still
lived. He even regarded his original Glasgow chair as a useful
stepping stone to get to London, 'my natural place'. If Glasgow
had been a stepping stone, then Edinburgh was to be a
launching pad.

On 10 February 1877, Sir William Fergusson, the Professor
of Surgery at King's College, London died. A caucus on the
College Council tried to persuade Lister to take his place, but
there was a problem: Lister insisted on continuing Syme's
method of clinical teaching – to lecture to students on live cases
in the operating theatre (rather than the lecture theatre) – and
this was not done in London.

The Edinburgh students got up a petition begging Lister to stay. He prevaricated, saying he would not go to London if he had 'to teach clinical surgery as it is taught in any London school at the present time'. But his clear insult to London teaching methods made it very difficult for King's to appoint him to succeed Fergusson: they would appear to be condoning his criticism.

So the Professorship of Surgery went elsewhere. Lister wrote to a friend 'it is finally decided that I am not going to King's . . . I find it easy to fall back on the belief that my position here is that in which I can best serve my generation.' His students were delighted.

But the King's College caucus had not given up. They managed to get carried a motion expressing a general desire that Lister become the Professor of *Clinical* Surgery, i.e. they proposed to create a new Chair specially for him, one which would enable him to teach just as he desired. Negotiations continued (Lister was certainly in London in May for a meeting of the General Medical Council) and on 6 June the Board of King's College Hospital gave their approval for the new post, and Lister was formally appointed to it on 18 June 1877. The Listers moved to London on 11 September.

His first public duty in London was to give an Introductory Address to his students, and he decided to talk on germ theory. His precious flasks and tubes of 'cultures' had been carefully brought to London from Edinburgh, resting on his and Mrs Lister's knees in the railway carriage. Now they were carefully transported by horse-drawn carriage to Somerset House. John Stewart, one of Lister's trainees, described the journey: 'We supported the trays and glasses as carefully as possible. They had been brought successfully all the way from Edinburgh, but were now in perilous passages, there were occasional awkward jolts and they sometimes rattled terribly. I made some remark about 'Caesar and his fortunes' and I well remember his gentle, amused and somewhat pensive smile.'[42]

Incidentally, Margaret Mathewson got it wrong when she wrote that Lister was moving to St Thomas's, it was to King's College, London. His successor as Professor of Clinical Surgery in Edinburgh was Thomas Annandale.

Margaret Mathewson   *Letter to her father, 18 October 1877*

. . . A Dr. Annandale has succeeded Professor Lister.
Tuesday afternoon he came downstairs and took down all
our names and said 'I want 8 empty beds tonight.' 4 were
turned out of bed and sent home as they were. Some got
lotion and dressing with them. Others got prescriptions
for to get it from the Druggist. (Some of them were crying
at being sent away unhealed.) Another 4 beds emptied in
No. 2 and some of his patients carried down stairs but the
4 empty beds is here yet. I was dressed in order to see if I
could be dismissed but its still not heal . . . Professor
Annandale has not looked at any of Professor Lister's
patients as yet but wants them all removed, either to other
wards or dismissed altogether and new Patients of his own
to take their places, and the wards is getting cleaned.
There is painters and 6 women going after them washing
the wood parts.

Sketch

. . . all Prof. Lister's patients were dismissed but Agnes
and I, and we two were divided. Agnes was put into
Dr. Bell's No. 1 ward, and I was kept in No. 3. There was
one patient who had been in 12 months, Lizzie Thomas.
She had been in bed all the time. Her wounds were not
quite healed, and she had to stay in bed 6 weeks after it
was healed. Thus Dr. Roxburgh telegraphed to London to
Prof. Lister if he could take this patient.
'Yes, and she must travel in bed.'

Letter to her family, 6 November 1877

. . . Miss Logan went to London with a female patient of
Professor Lister's. Arthur will have an idea who she is as
she was in the second bed on the left hand side from the
door and had a soras abscess in her left side. She got her
operation the following day she came in and was getting
on very well but still it was not healed up when Professor
Annandale came on duty . . . Annandale wanted all old

patients removed thus Dr Roxburgh wrote to London about her and Professor telegraphed back for her to be sent as soon as convenient but to travel in bed or in a lying position thus Miss Logan had to accompany her as special nurse and she was put into the operation basket and 6 students carried her to the station (and saw them off) and had some lark over it to the station as was no wonder for it was a singular instance and caused quite a commotion all through the Infirmary.

Lizzie Thomas was a parlour maid from Torquay who had been admitted to the Royal Infirmary on 1 August 1876, with a large psoas abscess (an abscess of the hip and spine) probably tubercular. John Stewart says she was: 'a very nice girl, and a great favourite on account of her cheerful patience'.

On Lister's departure, the Managers of the Infirmary decided that they had had enough of his long-stay patients, and Annandale did not want *his* record blemished by any of Lister's failures. So the chronic cases Lister had left behind were discharged. Stewart continues: 'I remember how his look of incredulity changed to one of sorrow and honest anger [when he heard] and he used the strongest expression I ever heard him utter. He said, "It's an infamous shame."'

When Stewart and Miss Logan arrived at King's College with their charge, Lizzie Thomas, the sister in charge would not let her in, because she had no proper admission papers. Stewart had to force his way in, with the help of the porter whose sense of honour he had touched: 'an old soldier like you can't stand and see a pretty girl lying on this stone-cold floor.' Lister performed a second operation on her in 1880, and she was alive and well in Torquay to greet Lister when he passed through in 1897.[43]

Lister moved his other chronic charges, six male patients, to an Edinburgh nursing home at his own expense. He also took William Watson Cheyne with him to London as his house surgeon.

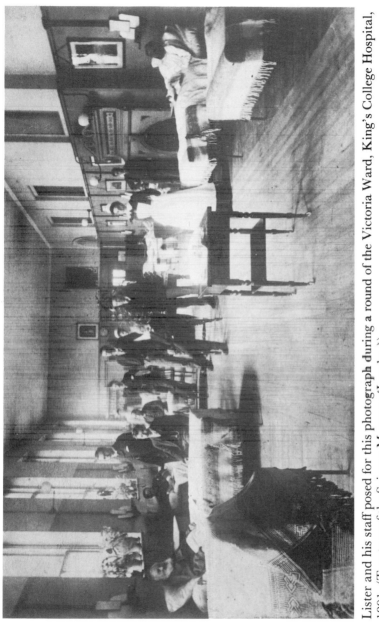

Lister and his staff posed for this photograph during a round of the Victoria Ward, King's College Hospital, 1891. (Trustees of the Science Museum (London))

In the spring of 1877 Lister received and ultimately accepted an invitation to go to London as Professor of Clinical Surgery at King's College. The first that I heard of it was one Sunday morning, I think a day or two after he received the invitation, when I was sleeping quietly in the house surgeon's bedroom. I woke up to find someone shaking me, and to my astonishment on opening my eyes I found that it was Lister. He told me about his invitation to London. He had not yet at all made up his mind about it, but if he went he would need to take a small staff with him familiar with his methods, and he had come down that morning to know whether, if he decided to go, I would go with him and again act as his house surgeon for six months at King's College Hospital. Go with Lister to London! I could not believe my ears! Of course I would go with him to London or anywhere else.[44]

DISCHARGE FROM HOSPITAL

William Ernest Henley

DISCHARGED in *Poems* (1898)

Carry me out
Into the wind and the sunshine,
Into the beautiful world.

O, the wonder, the spell of the streets!
The stature and strength of the horses,
The rustle and echo of footfalls,
The flat roar and rattle of wheels!
A swift tram floats huge on us . . .
It's a dream?
The smell of the mud in my nostrils
Blows brave – like a breath of the sea!

As of old,
Ambulant, undulant drapery,
Vaguely and strangely provocative,
Flutters and beckons. O, yonder –
Is it? – the gleam of a stocking!
Sudden, a spire

Wedged in the mist! O, the houses,
The long lines of lofty, grey houses,
Cross-hatched with shadow and light!
These are the streets . . .
Each is an avenue leading
Whither I will!

Free . . . !
Dizzy, hysterical, faint,

I sit, and the carriage rolls on with me
Into the wonderful world.

Margaret Mathewson   *Sketch*

I was dismissed 'cured' on October 23rd just 8 months to a
day since I entered. I went to Campbeltown to my brother
Walter. I stayed three weeks then went back to Edinburgh
on my way home to Shetland.

I had 2 days to wait for the Shetland boat, and so I
called up at the Infirmary as there might be any further
instructions regarding the dressing of my arm. Also I
wished to ask some questions regarding its treatment.
I saw Dr. Chiene. He did not recognize me at first.

'What was the operation?'

'Excision of the shoulder joint, sir.'

'Oh, that's a serious operation.' He looked at it and had
lots of questions. 'Certainly Professor Lister has made a
good job of you. You must have been a favourite case to
him – I now remember who you are. I was at your
operation.'

'Yes, sir.'

'Well, really you have progressed wonderfully, but
Prof. was very anxious about you when you were so sick
and had no hope of you getting over it.'

'Indeed, sir.'

'Yes, he went to the Infirmary 3 hours sooner than
usual, as he was fearing you would not be alive. It is really
a wonder how you have progressed. You can go home
safely now.'

'Thank you, sir.'

'Where is your home?'

'In Shetland.'

'How long does it take to go there?'

'Nearly a week, sir.'

'Dear-o-me that's nearly as long as it takes to go to
America. That's a long journey and you must take care of
your arm. It wants to be nursed. What do you dress it
with?'

'With Brassic lint and carbolic lotion, sir.'

140

'What's its strength?'

'From 1 to 40, sir.'

'That's rather strong now, but I will give you a prescription for Boric and Brassic ointment. Put that on Brassic lint and be sure and write me and let me know how it gets on.'

'Thank you, sir. But please sir what's your charge for advice?'

'Nothing at all as you have been such a long time in the Infirmary and now having to go so far North, I daresay you will need all your money.'

Letter to her brother Arthur, November 1877

Dear Brother,

I am resolved on going home per steamer and have brought my Box here and as I fancied you might be busy and therefore I wouldn't have an opportunity of speaking to you, I wrote this.

I got 16/– from home and I changed the stamps at the General and they kept 6d off and I bought a hat for 4/– and a hair net etc for the other 1/– so that only left 10/6d and I require 10/– for steamer; freight and 1/6d from Lerwick to Mid Yell and I would need some provision in the steamer with me. I'm sorry to be under the necessity to ask you for anything.

Meantime I am yours in haste.

Sketch

In the summer of '78 Dr. Cheyne (who went to London with Prof. Lister) came home for his holidays. I went to Fetlar to see him for advice on my arm also to let him see its progress. He probed it to see if it was sound at the bone. I felt it in the shoulder cup, and for some days after it was very sore. He asked if it had ever gathered.

'Yes sir it gathered three times after I came home.'

'What did you do?'

'I wrote Dr. Chiene, Edinburgh and he sent me a drainage tube.'

'And who put it in?'

'Myself, sir, before a glass.'

He was very much amused and surprised at this, then had lots of questions. Then he said: 'Well it is quite sound at the bone and it will doubtless get to be as strong as the other yet, and what a successful case it came to be and I am so glad to see it.'

It healed quite up in August and since feels much stronger. It was 17 months healing. Now I can do any sort of indoor work – even washing clothes etc. And looking back through this ordeal of trouble how I am led to wonder, and adore God's love and mercy who sustained me through it.

William Ernest Henley

TO R.T.H.B. in *Poems* (1898)

Out of the night that covers me,
Black as the Pit from pole to pole,
I thank whatever gods may be
For my unconquerable soul.

In the fell clutch of circumstance
I have no winced nor cried aloud.
Under the bludgeonings of chance
My head is bloody, but unbowed.

Beyond this place of wrath and tears
Looms but the Horror of the shade,
And yet the menace of the years
Finds, and shall find, me unafraid.

It matters not how strait the gate,
How charged with punishments the scroll,
I am the master of my fate:
I am the captain of my soul.

R.T.H.B. was R. T. Hamilton Bruce, one of Henley's (and Stevenson's) bourgeois Bohemian friends in Edinburgh. This poem was rather popular in the Edwardian era, when it was generally known as *Invictus*.

Henley left hospital some time in April 1875, and decided to stay on in Edinburgh: he became one of Robert Louis Stevenson's circle of friends: young men of the middle class who enjoyed dabbling their toes in the stream of hard-drinking, hard-living, working-class life that surged beneath Edinburgh's genteel façade. Henley found work as a 'hack' on the *Encyclopaedia Britannica*, but soon was able to write to Harry Nichols of some more authentic writing: 'In July there will appear, in the *Cornhill Magazine*, a remarkable paper: Hospital Outlines, Sketches and Portraits, by a friend of ours, which his name, I will not deceive you is, not Harris, but Henley. I hope you will invest a shilling.'

The nine guineas he received did not go far, and he and Stevenson collaborated on what they hoped would be a more profitable venture, playwriting. They wrote four plays together: *Deacon Brodie, Beau Austin, Admiral Guinea* and *Macaire*, but signally failed to impress the theatre-going public. Eventually the two men quarrelled bitterly, and parted (though the more affluent Stevenson continued, surreptitiously, to support Henley). When Stevenson came to write *Treasure Island*, he wrote that Henley's 'maimed masterfulness gave me the germ from which John Silver grew'.

Henley moved to London, and became the editor of the influential literary and political weekly, *The National Observer* and, shedding his Bohemianism, became a stalwart of the British Empire. At one point he was a contender to succeed Tennyson as Poet Laureate. He failed there, but in his editorial role nurtured many important writers: Yeats, Kipling and Wells amongst them.

His foot gave him continuous pain, and severely restricted his movements. (Wells described him after their first meeting as 'a magnificient torso set upon shrunken withered legs', and he found his presence similar to that of Franklin D. Roosevelt.) Henley died, prematurely aged and overweight in 1903, aged 53.

Margaret Mathewson returned to Yell, where she wrote up several copies of the *Sketch*. The one used in this book was completed on 27 September 1879. She was successful in her ambition to persuade her fellow-islanders that 'hospital' was no longer a dirty word. The parish of Mid Yell sent the sum of £2 9s to the Infirmary from 'a collection made in the parish per Rev. James Barclay' for the year 1878–9, the only time Mid Yell appears as a contributor to the Infirmary funds.[45] Shortly afterwards Margaret's primary infection – tuberculosis of the lungs – flared up again and she died on 28 September 1880 at the age of 32. Her death could not be 'certified' as Yell still did not have a doctor.

In his 'official' biography of Lister, Rickman Godlee wrote:

> Chronic cases of tuberculous disease of bone, complicated with abscesses, formerly almost invariably fatal, became curable [with Lister's operation plus antiseptic treatment]; but only by very prolonged and scrupulously careful treatment. To send them back to their homes before healing was complete was practically to send them to their deaths, or at best to condemn them to years of misery. But there was a danger of the wards becoming filled with such chronic cases to the exclusion of the more interesting and some would say more important acute cases.[46]

Margaret was *not* one of those patients immediately discharged by the hospital authorities on Lister's departure; she was given another fortnight. Admittedly, she wanted to leave and the turmoil that followed the arrival of the new professor, and the loss of friendly familiar faces, all helped to drive her out, but responsible doctors should have tried to persuade her to stay on at least a little longer.

Certainly in the harsh climate of the Shetlands, in a crowded and not particularly well-off household, and urged on by her work ethic, she would have had no respite.

The year 1880 was a tragic one for the Mathewson family. First Arthur died at the age of 41. His father wrote:

> After all that Mortals & Medicines could do My Beloved Arthur departed this life at 9.50 on the morning of Friday February 20th. Margaret has been in bed ever since.

For nearly the last twelve months almost all I could say of his recovery was the Proverb while there's life there's hope. I slept with him to the last two nights and had seen him often worse than he appeared to be that morning. Margaret and the lasses residing with us have often watched all night – Margaret who after her protracted sojurn in the Royal Infirmary Edinburgh was well prepared for every attention.

After that, it is perhaps not surprising that Margaret's illness returned. On 21 September, her brother Walter, the lighthouse keeper in Campbeltown, was expecting the worst: 'we was sorry to find that Sister Margaret was no better, but if anything weaker and that the purging still continues. I hope that if she can take what Mr. Barclay give her that it will be the means of stopping it, but if it should be otherwise I believe she is prepared for a happy exchange . . .'

Walter's letter continues: 'I also saw the Dr. and got a bottle from him to strengthen me; I am feeling better but my throat still continues a little swelled. The Cough is entirely away and my appetite some better, so if I once get on to eat well I will soon get stronger.'

It was not to be however, and he died on 31 October 1880, aged 38. Their father, Andrew Dishington Mathewson, was heartbroken: 'All three died in one year and I may say by one preventable disease – catching cold – which a little care and a little more clothes could easily have attended to.' In fact, it was almost certainly tuberculosis that killed all three.[47]

AFTERWORD

Most first-hand accounts of Lister have come from doctors who were his students, while those of Henley and Mathewson were written, as patients, much closer to the events. However, this does not mean that their accounts should be taken as impartial.

Henley's crushing weakness as a poet is insincerity. Too often his verses are written for calculated effect rather than stating genuine feelings and responses to events. This is most clearly seen in the Robert Louis Stevenson episode. When Stevenson writes that Henley was intoxicated by the beauty of the countryside in spring, having been incarcerated in a gloomy hospital for 18 months, that seems perfectly reasonable. In his poem 'Pastoral' Henley evidently decided it would not be sufficiently poetic to admit that he had been genuinely delighted, so a clanking downbeat final verse is added. (Some of his other poems have been edited to remove such verses.) In letters to a close friend, Henley might have been expected to be more honest, and certainly some of his sexual references have proved too explicit for his biographers, even for the 1949 biography. But these are the letters of a writer trying out effects for future poems; almost all are begging letters, ending up by asking Harry Nichols to send money.

Margaret Mathewson's *Sketch* is also biased. It is an evangelical tract and, as she writes in her preface, meant to convert people to hospitals and her brand of Methodism. In the conversations she reports with such vivacity, many of her interlocutors speak in planted phrases (perhaps difficult to avoid) and surely some in planted sentiments. Even when she has no axe to grind, she or the hospital grapevine can still get facts wrong, as when she thinks Lister is going to a Professorship at St Thomas's in London.

The conventional histories of Lister and antiseptics have, however, painted a far more distorted picture, one which is only now being rectified by medical historians. It is *not* true to say that all was dinginess, sepsis and suppuration before Lister, and then all became light. The situation was very much more complicated because, along with antiseptics, there occurred at least three other simultaneous revolutions: better nursing, increased cleanliness and improved nutrition.

Many of the nurses whom both Mathewson and Henley encountered in Edinburgh, Miss Logan for one, were 'Nightingales', namely nurses trained in Florence Nightingale's precepts either by her at St Thomas's Hospital, London or, at one remove, by Nightingale-trained nurses in Edinburgh.

Florence Nightingale was one of those remarkable individuals who *do* single-handedly change history. Before her, nursing was a generally despised profession. The unavoidable close proximity to the infectiously ill meant that only women who could no longer support themselves by any other means would turn to nursing. Florence Nightingale changed that. She came from a well-to-do family, but at the age of 17 (1837) she had a 'vision' calling her to nursing. The conflict between her calling and her family caused her a nervous breakdown, but she persevered. She was so successful in improving the standards of care in one of the small London hospitals in the early 1850s that the government asked her to go to the Crimean War to see what could be done there. She was horrified by the squalor and filth she found in military hospitals and her success in cleaning them up made her a national heroine. Nursing became a respectable *profession*; indeed the first opportunity for respectable women to have a career and independence. In 1860 she set up a nursing school at St Thomas's and was able to pick and choose qualified and motivated middle-class girls to train. Providing efficient, attentive, intelligent nurses in hospitals was one of her achievements and one of growing importance as medicine itself became more sophisticated and scientific. Also, according to R. B. Fisher, by providing all the nation's hospitals with nurses trained at a single centre, she forced on the doctors a standardization of medical terminology.

Florence Nightingale also contributed to the revolution in hospital hygiene. Part of her creed was cleanliness, soap and

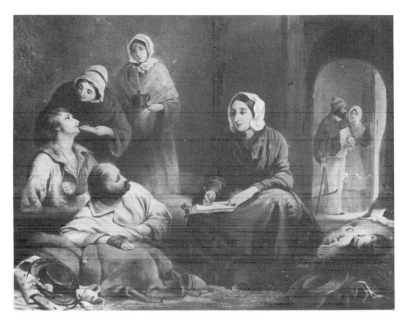

Above: The popular image of Florence Nightingale. (BBC Hulton Picture Library); *below:* Florence Nightingale learning about hospital design at Scutari. (BBC Hulton Picture Library)

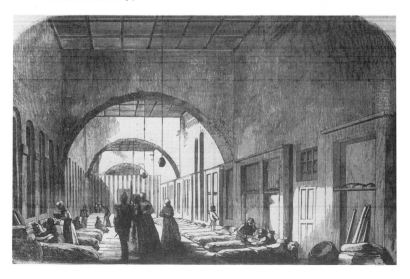

water. She had read Simpson and tried his statistical methods on 24 London hospitals, claiming, inaccurately in fact, that 90.84 per cent of their patients died in 1861. None the less, she believed that cleanliness was at least part of the answer. Some sort of theoretical justification was made from the observation that in the bad (sulphurous) air of the city, washing a silver spoon in cold water delayed tarnishing: thus in the 'bad' air of the hospitals might sepsis be prevented by washing? Better still, Syme had tried wiping his hands and scalpels on a clean towel before starting to operate and claimed it was effective.

Florence Nightingale investigated the situation in the wards and in 1854 she wrote:

> Nurses did not as a general rule wash patients, they could *never* wash their feet – and it was with difficulty and only in great haste that they could have a drop of water, just to *dab* their hands and face. The beds on which the patients lay were dirty. It was common practice to put a new patient into the same sheets used by the last occupant of the bed, and mattresses were generally flock-sodden and seldom if ever cleaned.[48]

In antiquated hospital buildings, such as those in the Edinburgh Royal Infirmary where, for example, there were no bathrooms (see p. 25), the Nightingales had a running battle to keep dirt at bay. Margaret Mathewson wrote in her *Sketch*:

> On Saturday evening Nurse McConnachy came after supper and asked, 'Who wants their feet washed here?'
> We all said, 'I do nurse please.'
> 'Well all that's walking about will go to the scullery and wash their own, take soap and towels with you from the towel drawer and I will wash all that's in bed.'
> This was done every Saturday night and all the children bathed every Tuesday and Friday. The beds were changed, also our body clothes and there was a washing house and 12 washerwomen in it daily, also a washing machine, and most of the clothes were steam dried. The patients were allowed to put one bed gown and chemise to each washing. We had a private mark into each article.

Hospital administrators, too, had read Simpson's work. If bad air was causing 'hospitalism', perhaps it could be overcome by dilution, by decreasing the number of patients per hospital ward (or as Godlee put it 'more cubic feet were allotted to each bed') and by improving ventilation.

When it was decided that the buildings of the Edinburgh Royal Infirmary were no longer adequate, a decision made in 1870 after six years of debate, the architect asked Florence Nightingale's advice about the design of wards for adequate ventilation and sanitation. The 'pavilion' ward she recommended was adopted and proved to be highly successful when the new building was opened in 1879.

The authorities in Glasgow prided themselves on their efforts to deal with their hospital's ventilation, even though they had to cope with a city whose population was rapidly expanding. They were outraged when Lister wrote: 'I was engaged in a perpetual contest with the managing body, who, anxious to provide hospital accommodation for the increasing population were disposed to introduce additional beds.' The authorities replied that they had *not* increased the number of beds, but kept them static at 144[49]. It is rather ironic that Lister should have chosen this point on which to belabour Glasgow's managers, for under similar pressure he had coped if anything rather worse. When word of his 'miracle' treatment had been passed around, heart-breaking cases from all over the country (from Shetland and Margate, for example) had presented themselves to him, and rather than turn them away he had grossly overcrowded his wards. This overcrowding was only exacerbated by his prolonged use of carbolic therapy.

If Glasgow's hospital authorities found it difficult to deal with overcrowding, her civic authorities were made of sterner stuff. William Tennant Gairdner, a colleague of Lister at the Royal Infirmary, became the first part-time Medical Officer of Health in 1863. He was assisted by five part-time District Surgeons of Police, and his job was to make the city healthier. He was given extraordinary powers, including that of 'ticketing'. He could post a notice outside a house showing the maximum number of occupants the house was allowed. In 1870 the police carried out 47,163 raids to ensure the 'tickets' were complied with. By preventing overcrowding in houses, just as in hospitals, he hoped that the spread of disease would be halted. By promoting sanitation schemes, he hoped that disease would not even get started.[50]

To keep the city, its people and its hospitals clean required volumes of clean water. This in itself became possible only after the middle of the nineteenth century. Glasgow, for example, had always relied on wells and the Clyde, but by the beginning of the nineteenth century, as the population increased, both sources became polluted. Glasgow's inhabitants increasingly found themselves drinking their own sewage.

Private companies were set up to bring water in, either through pipes or in wooden barrels to be sold in the streets. The piped water often failed in dry spells and never got to the higher points of the city at all, and even if the wooden barrels could be trundled to places the pipes could not reach, this water was expensive and it was hard work carrying buckets of water up flights of stairs to the tops of tenements. In either case water was a valuable commodity, to be used for such essential purposes as extending the life of a bottle of whisky, but *not* for inessentials such as washing.

The importance of an adequate supply of water was realized (for hard-headed industrial reasons, as well as domestic ones) but plans to provide such a supply were thwarted by the water companies' political chicanery, and the expense of the new scheme, which would have to be borne by ratepayers.

It took 30 years before civic resolve, pride and finance won through, and then only after three major outbreaks of cholera, in 1832, 1848 and 1853. By then, the evidence linking cholera to polluted water was hardening: when the civic officials of Edinburgh asked the Prime Minister, Palmerston, to proclaim a national day of fasting and humiliation in the hope of divine intervention to halt the epidemic of 1853, Palmerston told them rather to build drains and toilets.

In 1855 work started on a grandiose scheme to turn Loch Katrine into Glasgow's municipal reservoir. Some 25 miles of aqueduct were driven by hammer, steel and blasting powder through 'the most obdurate material' by a workforce of 2,000 men. By the autumn of 1859 the aqueduct was finished, and on 14 October Queen Victoria raised the sluice which turned on Glasgow's water.

Punch was ready with a little poem:

Glasca's just a'richt the noo,
She has got Loch Katrine brought her;
Ever she had the mountain dew,
Noo she rins wi' mountain water.
Hech the blessin'! ho the boon!
Tae ilka drouthie Glesca body,
Sin' there's water in the toon
Owre eneuch to mak its toddie.

Glesca chiels, a truth ye'll learn,
New to mony a Scot, I'm thinkin';
Water, aiblins, ye'll discern
Was na gi'en alane for drinkin',
Hauns and face ye'll scrub at least
Frae ane until anither Monday,
Gif nae Sabbatarian beast
Stap your Waterworks on Sunday.

The fact that clean fresh water could suddenly be commanded in the middle of a tenement *did* bring about a revolution in cleanliness, even if, for some of those more set in their ways, it took some getting used to. One old lady, who all her life had used a local well, complained bitterly when the authorities decided to close it down because of pollution. 'Hoots woman, why need you fash yoursel,' advised a well-meaning neighbour, 'you've got gravitation water in the hoose.' 'Huh, I just cannot thole that new water, its got neither taste nor smell.'

Punch may have had a superior snigger at Glasgow's expense but Glasgow had the belly laugh; by 1860, the year Lister moved to the city, her people and industry had abundant clean water while London was still drinking the raw Thames.

The third concurrent revolution was dietary. This is much more difficult to confirm than the others, but recent work has shown that there was an increase in the 'real' standard of living around the middle of the nineteenth century in Glasgow; wages rose and employment became more secure. This rise in the standard of living meant that people could afford more and better food (and to prepare it better with the 'gravitation'

153

water). The general health of the population improved. One indication of this was a reduction in the number of people admitted to hospital suffering from illnesses such as typhus and leg ulcers, generally indicators of a poor standard of living. The natural resistance of people to infectious disease and, inside hospital, to postoperative infection must also have simultaneously improved.[51]

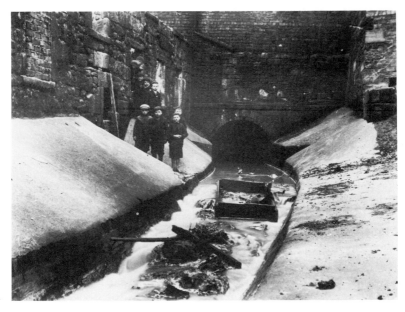

Glasgow children paddling barefoot in raw sewage, c. 1910. It took a long time for the basic notions of hygiene to sink in. (Strathclyde Regional Archives)

Lister's antiseptic surgery must therefore be seen in context. It happened at a time when *all* patients in hospitals were receiving better attention from properly trained nurses; at a time when hospital authorities were trying to make hospitals more hygienic, when civic authorities were making cities cleaner and when purer water supplies were beginning; and at a time

154

when the population was becoming substantially healthier through better nutrition. Thus antiseptics joined the crest of an established wave.

In fact, the evangelistic fervour of the antiseptics 'movement' blinded many of its converts to its faults. Lister knew the importance of the body's natural defences: during his series of compound fracture cases, he lectured to his students: 'it is never Man that heals a disease; it is always Nature: all that man can do is to remove obstacles.' On another occasion he wrote: 'we must destroy in the first instance once and for all any septic organisms which may exist within the part concerned; and after this has been done our efforts must be directed to the prevention of others into it. And provided these indications are *really* fulfilled, the less the antiseptic agent comes in contact with the living tissue the better.'

And here, precisely, lay the problem. Carbolic acid is not specific: as well as killing germs it kills the cells of the body, the cells of the skin around the wound and white blood cells, the body's natural defence against invading germs. Thus carbolic acid and all the other antiseptics of the day not only sterilized the surgeon's hands and instruments before an operation, which was without doubt beneficial, but also killed many of the body's own cells and lowered its resistance, which was detrimental. Indeed, even while Lister was developing antiseptic surgery, other surgeons, following and developing Syme's precepts of cleanliness in the operating theatre, were far more successful than Lister with this regimen. Some seem to have achieved lower mortality figures with soap and water alone than Lister did with antiseptics.

The most notable of these was Thomas Keith, who worked alongside Lister in Edinburgh. He was scrupulous in his attentions to cleanliness, using distilled water to wash his patients and boiling his surgical sponges before each operation. Many of the surgeons who disliked the antiseptic 'movement' rushed to cite Keith's work as proof that Lister's regimen was unnecessary. Keith, however, was a friend and defender of Lister: the development of his style of treatment probably owed a lot to Lister's *analysis* of the cause of sepsis.

None the less, Lister really should have paid much closer attention to Keith's work than he did. Instead, he continued to drench everything in carbolic. He eventually recognized that the steam spray was a waste of time and abandoned it, but he never changed his basic tenets. Once he had failed with cleanliness and cold water he never doubted its uselessness and, in fact, became a less painstaking surgical operator after the introduction of carbolic (see p. 69). He even disapproved when Cheyne began using rubber surgical gloves, because he thought that any improvement in hygiene might distract doctors' attention from the importance of carbolic.

All this seems very odd if one looks at the very beginnings of the antiseptic movement. The first time carbolic is mentioned in Lister's Ward Books was on 10 December 1864, in the treatment of Andrew Connel, a nine-year-old boy with a tuberculous wrist:

> For the last two days the sores have been dressed with Carbolic Acid, the day before yesterday the acid was used with about an equal part of water, and had the effect of entirely preventing fetor, and almost entirely preventing suppuration; yesterday it was used 1–16 which has been followed by some purulent discharge, though small in quantity but distinctly fetid. Similar effects were produced in three other cases in which the Carbolic Acid has been used during the same period; in one case that of Mary Ann Lavander (wrist joint) the weaker solution entirely prevented suppuration from a considerable sore and without causing the uneasiness that the stronger proportions did. On the whole, however, it cannot be said that cicatrization [the formation of healthy scar tissue] has made satisfactory progress under it; on the contrary the newly developed epidermis seems rather to have been destroyed by the Carbolic Acid, which would seem to act with special facility on the epidermis; the surface of the granulations in some cases appear to have become slightly excavated under it, at the same time not the slightest redness has been produced on the neighbouring skin.
> The sulphite has been therefore returned to. In one other case however an amputation of the ankle accompanied with considerable suppuration and fetor, the powerful antiseptic properties of the Carbolic Acid were of such conspicuous advantage that it has been continued.[52]

Carbolic was clearly no 'wonder drug', and its main disadvantage was visible from the beginning.

Furthermore, it is clear that Lister had not yet heard of germs when he began using carbolic. Godlee is quite definite that it was not until 1865 that Anderson first told Lister of Pasteur's work. Also, the description of Thomas Murdoch's death from hospital gangrene (see p. 9), probably caught from a patient in the next bed, occurred three months after the use of carbolic had begun. Yet no mention of the possibility of cross-infection is made in Murdoch's case notes nor, more significantly, was any effort made to isolate the already gangrenous patient. It is difficult to believe that Lister could have really accepted Pasteur's ideas and yet allowed this to happen. The treatment of Charles Cobb's compound fracture (see p. 12) using, effectively, aseptic techniques a fortnight before Murdoch's admission must therefore have been fortuitous. Carbolic acid was, at least to begin with, merely an addition to the list of available disinfectants. Indeed, potassium sulphite clearly remained the disinfectant of choice.*

---

* The year 1865 is given in R. Godlee, *Lord Lister*, third edition (Oxford, 1924), p. 162. This runs against the standard antiseptic myth, which Lister himself began in his famous *Lancet* paper (16 March 1867, p. 327), where he wrote:

> . . . Bearing in mind that it is from the vitality of the atmospheric particles that all the mischief arises, it appears that all that is requisite is to dress the wound with some material capable of killing these septic germs, provided that any substance can be found reliable for this purpose, yet not too potent as a caustic.
>
> In the course of the year 1864 I was much struck with an account of the remarkable effects produced by carbolic acid upon the sewage of the town of Carlisle . . .

This is misleading: he should have written 'In the course of the year 1864 I *had been* much struck . . .'. Godlee, having seen the year 1864 in this paper, and knowing that 1865 was the year Lister first heard of Pasteur, should have done better than to write (p. 182):

> . . . looking round for a suitable antiseptic, he remembered that he had heard of the way in which carbolic acid had been used as a disinfectant in dealing with the sewage at Carlisle, and the striking results which had been obtained.

Pages of Lister's Glasgow Ward Book for 1864 with the first record of the use of carbolic acid. (Archives, University of Glasgow)

Andrew Cornue, cont.d 222.

The Scaphoid was a mere shell, some of the metacarpal bones were also affected and the cartilage of the radius was thin and rough. He suffered pain the first night, but in the morning was easy, already he could move the finger and the thumb freely. The dressing was removed so far this, the Ulnar incision was explored and a poultice applied

28th Nov

Last night was restless but today he is smiling and easy; the movement of the fingers as yesterday. A little passive movement of fingers and thumb performed. The hand is at present suffering from an aggravation of the swelling, dry lint removed and a poultice applied

By H. Carter

29th Nov

His bowels have been acted on by the 2 Pisine, which he got yesterday, & passed an easy night, though he did not get much sleep. The movement of the fingers and thumb are as perfect as it was yesterday, being able to stretch them completely today, & the second piece of lint has been removed this morning from the Ulnar incision. The swelling of the hand continues and there is a redness extending half way up the back of the forearm. Fingers freed. Poultice continued

p. 224.

30th Nov/64

Took a good breakfast and had a good night's rest. Only one superficial ligature was open at the operation

3d Decr/64

Yesterday it was dressed with dry lint; poultice discontinued; sore under the wrist diminishing and looking well; strips of plaster were applied over the radial incision.

6th Decr/64

Brings the thumb easily in contact with the second joint of the forefinger

10th Decr

The hand being unsupported the knuckles droop only very slightly below the horizontal level.

For the last few days the sores have been dressed with Carbolic acid, the day before yesterday the acid was pure with about an equal part of water, and had the effect of entirely preventing fetor, and almost entirely preventing suppuration, yesterday it was pure 1 16 which has been followed by some free discharge, though small in quantity but distinctly fetid. Similar effects were produced in three other cases in which the Carbolic acid has been used during the same period; in one case that of Mary Ann Lavander (wrist joint) the weather preventing acid entirely preventing suppuration

p. 225.

159

Diluting the concentration of the carbolic was no answer to its drawbacks, despite the hopeful comments made in Andrew Connel's case notes. In his textbook *Antiseptic Surgery*, published in 1882, W. W. Cheyne explores this matter further. He compared the different antiseptics available, and carbolic came out rather badly:

> And so my own experience of carbolic acid as a disinfectant in the form of a 1–40 watery solution in putrid cases is unfavourable, while, on the other hand if 1–20 carbolic acid be used, it is very irritating, and interferes with healing. Injected once or twice a day, the latter destroys the superficial granulation cells, and produces a thin slough in which bacteria develop, and from which it is very difficult to dislodge them. Then its poisonous properties are objectionable . . . Hence I do not like carbolic acid unless it is used aseptically.

The best disinfectant *still* seemed to be sulphurous acid:

> This is a powerful germicide. It is also non-irritating and perfectly free from any poisonous qualities.

This was written *after* the antiseptic revolution.

Cheyne is very clear on the distinction between aseptic and antiseptic surgery, emphasizing that Lister's aim was really to *prevent* germs establishing themselves in wounds, rather than killing them once they were already there. For this purpose, in his opinion, carbolic acid for washing hands and surgical instruments and for filling the spray was a good thing. But no one, it seems, ever tried spraying any of the *other* antiseptics available and, despite its drawbacks, Lister based his antiseptic revolution on carbolic.

Perhaps, unconsciously, he was being a rather good politician. If he tried to sell the revolutionary idea of germs and aseptic surgery to other surgeons he knew opposition would be immense, particularly if he said that the treatment was to use a standard established chemical, albeit in a novel way. To convince other surgeons he had to slip his new ideas in on the back of a new treatment, and slip that in on the back of a new chemical. Surgeons were practical men; it was easier to sell them hardware than novel ideas. If, later, he became a devout believer in carbolic, not bothering to change or wash his surgical gown, he was not the first case in history of a man converted by his own rhetoric. It was left to other surgeons, particularly German ones and Lister's pupil in Glasgow, Sir William MacEwen, to develop a consistent aseptic regimen once the germ theory was established. The operating theatre and the surgeon's gowns, gloves and instruments were made sterile, the patient's skin around the site of surgery was treated with anti-septic, but after the operation the body's natural defences were left to deal with invading germs (whose entry to the wound had been rendered as unlikely as possible).

The real poverty of antiseptic surgery (and aseptic, too) was revealed in the First World War. There, in the tents that served as hospitals, in the mud and slime of the trenches, it was difficult to maintain the sterile conditions necessary for aseptic surgery. Furthermore, many of the wounded soldiers had lain in no man's land for days before being rescued and arrived at the hospitals with heavily infected wounds. Obviously, if sepsis was already under way, 'aseptic' surgery was not possible and carbolic acid had to be used. But on those wounds where suppuration was well established it proved to be more or less useless. Here, at least, it did nothing more than provide a culture medium for germs. Ironically, often the most severely wounded soldiers fared best. When these soldiers were left alone and unconscious their wounds would become infected with maggots, and the maggots in general did a better job than the surgeon. They ate the dead and decaying flesh, excreting a mild antibiotic, alantoin, and so providing less of a substrate for the invasion of germs. But to conscious soldiers their tickling was unbearable.

By the end of the war surgeons had developed a technique to imitate the maggots, called 'deep suture', where all the damaged flesh was cut away around the wound (almost regard-less of what organs had been damaged) and the patient then sewn up.

It was the first-hand experience of the carnage wrought by surgeons in the First World War that inspired Alexander Fleming to seek a new *specific* antiseptic that would kill germs and leave human cells unaffected, a search which led to penicillin and the host of modern antibiotic agents.

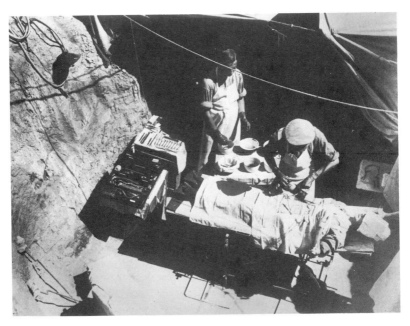

Field surgery in the First World War. Inside the tents there was no light or ventilation; outside there were dust and flies. (Wellcome Institute Library, London)

Yet even if antiseptic surgery was a failure in its strictest interpretation, Lister was undoubtedly a very great man, for he brought science back to medicine. Although his spray was less effective than he supposed, his clinical trials of different antiseptics – first on himself, then on his patients – helped introduce the experimental method into surgery. He developed a better 'catgut' for surgical stitching by carefully pickling sheep's intestines (the raw ingredient of catgut) in antiseptics of varying concentrations for varying periods, and then trying them out on animals. The fact that he was a scientist explains, in part, his charisma:

> Another unique characteristic was his habit of lecturing upon his mistakes. The architect is unfortunate in that his errors endure and testify to his limitations, but the doctor buries his failures; professional mistakes are usually regarded as legitimate objects for defence, and awaken ancient reflexes of self-preservation which beginning in the nursery follow to the school and usually persist throughout life, and 'not guilty' is ever upon our lips! You can imagine, then, the astonishment when one day at the close of a lecture Lister quietly announced that at our next meeting he would lecture upon the mistake he had made the day before.
>
> It was a bad case of goitre and the removal of the diseased gland had lately been attempted; the operation was new and there was little experience to guide, the method being that of simple excision of the growth. The haemorrhage was appalling and the patient died. Lister was deeply moved: he had not contemplated disaster, and on reflection it occurred to him that had he ligatured the thyroid arteries before he removed the gland, a life might have been saved.
>
> I remember his pathetic remorse and how he blamed himself for his want of caution. He told us he had read up the anatomy before the operation, but was quite unprepared for the deluge of blood, and that in future he should ligature every vessel before the removal of the gland. Plaintively he impressed upon us the importance of always studying our mistakes and never glossing them over, and of pointing out to others where we had gone wrong and so avoiding a repetition.[53]

If Lister's habit of calling his patients 'experiments' to their faces seemed callous, it was in some sense necessary, for he was trying to break centuries of malpractice and establish surgery on a scientific basis.

And many of his operations were experimental: even the application of antiseptic techniques to an old-established operation was in a sense an experiment. The excisions he performed on Henley and Mathewson were not 'new' operations, in that others had excised tubercular joints before, but to find the best way to excise a joint under an antiseptic regimen *was* a new operation. Being a perfectionist, Lister was never convinced that he had found an optimum procedure. Cheyne wrote, 'It would be hopeless to attempt to give any sort of list of the new operations which Lister did, and he himself absolutely declined to publish them.'[54]

Lister was perfectly aware of the change he was bringing to surgery. In Glasgow he had worked hard to ensure that students coming to read medicine had a more thorough scientific grounding. He always believed German doctors were quick to appreciate antiseptic surgery because of the better education they had received. Part of his insistence on clinical teaching in London was to get his students when they were young and impressionable and imbue them with scientific surgery.

On his move to King's College, London, in 1877, the *Medical Examiner* wrote that to the 'stronghold of the surgery of action' they were bringing 'the apostle of the surgery of thought'. That contemporary tribute makes a very just appreciation of Lister's real importance.

REFERENCES

1 J. R. Leeson, *Lister as I Knew Him* (London, 1927), p. 4.
2 J. Duns, *Memoir of Sir J. Y. Simpson* (Edinburgh, 1873), p. 231.
3 J. Duns, *Memoir of Sir J. Y. Simpson,* p. 258.
4 R. Godlee, *Lord Lister,* third edition (Oxford, 1924), p. 132.
5 R. Godlee, *Lord Lister,* p. 137.
6 R. Godlee, *Lord Lister,* p. 136–7.
7 R. B. Fisher, *Joseph Lister* (London, 1977), p. 126.
8 Ward Book 126, Glasgow University Medical Archive, pp. 285–9.
9 J. R. Leeson, *Lister as I Knew Him,* p. 94.
10 Ward Book 126, Glasgow University Medical Archive, p. 275.
11 Ward Book 126, Glasgow University Medical Archive, pp. 280–1.
12 K. Williamson, *W. E. Henley* (London, 1930), p. 29.
13 W. E. Henley, undated letter of 1872 to Harry Nichols in Huntingdon Library, Pasadena.
14 J. Connell, *W. E. Henley* (London, 1949), p. 47.
15 K. Williamson, *W. E. Henley,* pp. 29–30; see also L. Cope Cornford, *W. E. Henley* (London, 1913), pp. 25–6.
16 J. Graham, *New Shetlander,* vol. 39, p. 17, and personal communication.
17 J. T. Reid, *Art Rambles in Shetland* (Edinburgh, 1869), pp. 32–3.
18 D. Hamilton, *The Healers: a History of Scottish Medicine* (Edinburgh, 1981), pp. 173–4.
19 W. B. Howie and S. A. B. Black, *British Medical Journal,* vol. 2 (1976), pp. 515–17.
20 R. B. Fisher, *Joseph Lister,* p. 207.
21 Edinburgh Royal Infirmary Archives.

22 R. Shields, *Cornhill Magazine* (1905), pp. 223–7.
23 J. R. Leeson, *Lister as I Knew Him*, pp. 137–8.
24 F. Caird in *Joseph Baron Lister* (London, 1927), pp. 135–6.
25 R. B. Fisher, *Joseph Lister*, p. 64.
26 R. J. S. McDowall, *The Whiskies of Scotland*, third edition (London, 1975), p. 117.
27 R. B. Fisher, *Joseph Lister*, pp. 131, 210.
28 R. B. Fisher, *Joseph Lister*, p 106.
29 J. R. Leeson, *Lister as I Knew Him*, pp. 154–5.
30 A. Conan Doyle, *Round the Red Lamp*, second edition (London, 1934), pp. 9–19.
31 A. Conan Doyle, *Memories and Adventures*, second edition (London, 1930), p. 33.
32 D. Hamilton, *The Healers*, p. 227.
33 R. B. Fisher, *Joseph Lister*, pp. 207–8.
34 Ward Book 126, Glasgow University Medical Archive, pp. 137–8.
35 R. B. Fisher, *Joseph Lister*, p. 193.
36 R. Godlee, *Lord Lister*, p. 305.
37 R. Shields, *Cornhill Magazine* (1905), pp. 223–7.
38 D. Hamilton, *The Healers*, p. 96.
39 F. W. Maitland, *The Life and Letters of Leslie Stephen* (London, 1906), pp. 250–1.
40 S. Colvin, *Letters of R. L. Stevenson*, second edition (London, 1900), pp. 86–7.
41 S. Colvin, *Letters of R. L. Stevenson*, p. 94.
42 R. Godlee, *Lord Lister*, p. 414.
43 R. Godlee, *Lord Lister*, p. 412.
44 W. W. Cheyne, *Lister and his Achievement* (London, 1925), p. 31.
45 Edinburgh Royal Infirmary Archives.
46 R. Godlee, *Lord Lister*, p. 411.
47 J. Graham, personal communication.
48 R. B. Fisher, *Joseph Lister*, p. 126.
49 R. B. Fisher, *Joseph Lister*, p. 173.
50 D. Hamilton, *The Healers*, pp. 203–7.
51 D. Hamilton, *Bulletin of the History of Medicine*, vol. 56 (1982), pp. 30–40.
52 Ward Book 126, Glasgow University Medical Archive, pp. 222–5.

53 J. R. Leeson, *Lister as I Knew Him*, pp. 63–4.
54 W. W. Cheyne, *Lister and his Achievement*, p. 29.